SUBSTANCE ABUSE ASSESSMENT, INTERVENTIONS AND TREATMENT

STRENGTHENING THE SUBSTANCE USE TREATMENT WORKFORCE AND PROVIDER NETWORKS

SUBSTANCE ABUSE ASSESSMENT, INTERVENTIONS AND TREATMENT

Additional books in this series can be found on Nova's website under the Series tab.

Additional E-books in this series can be found on Nova's website under the E-book tab.

SUBSTANCE ABUSE ASSESSMENT, INTERVENTIONS AND TREATMENT

STRENGTHENING THE SUBSTANCE USE TREATMENT WORKFORCE AND PROVIDER NETWORKS

VALENTIN LEBLANC
EDITOR

nova publishers
New York

For permission to use material from this book please contact us:
Telephone 631-231-7269; Fax 631-231-8175
Web Site: http://www.novapublishers.com

Library of Congress Cataloging-in-Publication Data

ISBN: 978-1-62808-683-6

Published by Nova Science Publishers, Inc. † New York

CONTENTS

PREFACE

In 2004, over 23 million Americans age 12 and older needed specialty treatment for alcohol or illicit drug problems. Of those in need, only 10 percent received treatment at a specialty facility. There are a number of factors that contribute to low treatment participation rates. One of the most fundamental is the lack of an adequate human infrastructure to support current and future demands for treatment. The addictions treatment field is facing a workforce crisis. Worker shortages, inadequate compensation and stigma currently challenge the field. Increasingly, treatment and recovery support providers also struggle with issues related to recruitment, retention and professional development of staff. The ability to provide quality addictions treatment and recovery support services is severely hampered by these conditions. Without investment in human infrastructure, this critical public health function will not be equipped to respond effectively to the overwhelming need for services. This book includes a discussion of both long-term and emergent issues impacting the addictions treatment workforce and provides a context for understanding the challenges facing the addictions treatment workforce and a background for the recommendations that follow.

Chapter 1 - S*trengthening Professional Identity: Challenges of the Addictions Treatment Workforce* summarizes trends in addictions treatment and the challenges that confront the treatment workforce. Importantly, it also articulates a vision for the treatment and recovery support workforce by presenting a series of recommendations aimed at strengthening the field's professional identity. The recommendations in this report reflect some of the best thinking in the field and are intended to provide momentum for ongoing discussions among stakeholders about specific implementation strategies. The report discusses current trends in funding, staff recruitment and retention, patient characteristics and clinical practice and identifies recommendations in the following six areas: infrastructure, leadership and management, recruitment, education and accreditation, retention and studies priorities. *Strengthening Professional Identity* focuses on all professionals who provide addictions treatment and recovery support services, e.g., addictions counselors, physicians, psychologists, nurses, outreach and intake workers, case managers, social workers, marriage and family therapists, recovery support workers and clergy.

Chapter 2 - This study illustrates nine successful alcohol and other drug (AOD) addiction provider networks that are highly diverse in size, scope, complexity, and service array. These case studies are vignettes of the origins, current operations, strengths, and challenges of these networks. The reader will see how these organizations mounted strategies to address problems and challenges that are common throughout the addictions system.

The addictions treatment provider system is confronted with a variety of challenges in today's environment, including shrinking resources, increasing demands to demonstrate outcomes, patients with complex sets of problems calling for increased staff skills, and changes in business practices. These and other factors place high demands on the addictions treatment system. Small providers are especially hard-hit, unsure if they can continue to exist in this current environment, but large providers are not immune from the same struggles. Recruitment, retention, and professional development of staff are ongoing challenges to the field. Staff turnover rates in some areas are said to rival those in the fast-food industry. To survive and grow, agencies must find new methods of collaborating in order to maximize resources, retain staff, find strength and stability in a changing marketplace, and provide higher quality services based on sound and appropriate evidence-based practices. In a report entitled "Strengthening Professional Identity: Challenges of the Addictions Treatment Workforce", it is recommended that network strategies be fostered in order to strengthen the infrastructure of agencies and sustain the workforce.

Although networks and collaboration are not new concepts, it is important to examine various types of collaborations for strategies and structures that can strengthen and support providers. Lessons that might be learned from these organizations may be replicated in other communities. Some of the challenges in one part of the country are truly not that different in other regions. This report provides a unique opportunity to look at how other communities brought solutions to these common problems.

In: Strengthening …
Editor: Valentin LeBlanc
ISBN: 978-1-62808-683-6

Chapter 1

STRENGTHENING PROFESSIONAL IDENTITY: CHALLENGES OF THE ADDICTIONS TREATMENT WORKFORCE*

A FRAMEWORK FOR DISCUSSION

Melanie Whitter, E. Lorraine Bell, Peter Gaumond, Margaret Gwaltney, Candy A. Magaña and Mirabelle Moreaux

NOTE: The authors don't work for the government.

EXECUTIVE SUMMARY

In 2004, over 23 million Americans age 12 and older needed specialty treatment for alcohol or illicit drug problems. Of those in need, only 10 percent received treatment at a specialty facility (NSDUH, 2005). There are a number of factors that contribute to low treatment participation rates. One of the most fundamental is the lack of an adequate human infrastructure to support current and future demands for treatment. The addictions treatment field is facing a workforce crisis. Worker shortages, inadequate compensation

* This report was released by the Substance Abuse and Mental Health Services Administration, Partners for Recovery Initiative, December 2006.

and stigma currently challenge the field. Increasingly, treatment and recovery support providers also struggle with issues related to recruitment, retention and professional development of staff. The ability to provide quality addictions treatment and recovery support services is severely hampered by these conditions. Without investment in human infrastructure, this critical public health function will not be equipped to respond effectively to the overwhelming need for services.

Strengthening Professional Identity: Challenges of the Addictions Treatment Workforce summarizes trends in addictions treatment and the challenges that confront the treatment workforce. Importantly, it also articulates a vision for the treatment and recovery support workforce by presenting a series of recommendations aimed at strengthening the field's professional identity. The recommendations in this report reflect some of the best thinking in the field and are intended to provide momentum for ongoing discussions among stakeholders about specific implementation strategies. The report discusses current trends in funding, staff recruitment and retention, patient characteristics and clinical practice and identifies recommendations in the following six areas: infrastructure, leadership and management, recruitment, education and accreditation, retention and studies priorities. *Strengthening Professional Identity* focuses on all professionals who provide addictions treatment and recovery support services, e.g., addictions counselors, physicians, psychologists, nurses, outreach and intake workers, case managers, social workers, marriage and family therapists, recovery support workers and clergy.

Background and Approach

Workforce development has been an area of concern for the Substance Abuse and Mental Health Services Administration (SAMHSA) and for the addictions treatment field for many years. In recognition of the mounting workforce crisis, SAMHSA elevated workforce development to a program priority on its "SAMHSA Priorities: Programs and Principles Matrix." This designation has increased focus on this critical issue. The development of this stakeholder report began with an environmental scan of the recent research related to the treatment workforce.

Following the environmental scan, SAMHSA convened 128 individuals representing diverse stakeholder groups in nine separate stakeholder meetings from January through May 2004. During these meetings, SAMHSA solicited information and recommendations from representatives knowledgeable about the exceptional challenges faced by the addictions treatment workforce. Individuals from the following organizations and employment categories provided input: addictions counselors, Addiction Technology Transfer Centers (ATTCs), certification boards, Federal agencies, professional trade associations, clinical supervisors, college and university professors, faith-based providers, human resource managers, marriage and family therapists, nurses, physicians, psychiatrists, recovery support personnel, researchers, social workers, and State Directors. The participating Federal government partners represented a wide range of agencies, including the Departments of Labor, Transportation, Defense (Marine Corps and Navy), Veterans Affairs, Justice and Education, as well as the National Institute on Drug Abuse, the National Institute on Alcohol Abuse and Alcoholism, the Health Resources and Services Administration, the Centers for Medicare and Medicaid Services, and each of the SAMHSA Centers.

Context: Trends Impacting the Workforce

This report begins with a discussion of both long-term and emergent issues impacting the addictions treatment workforce. The information included in this section provides a context for understanding the challenges facing the addictions treatment workforce and a background for the recommendations that follow.

Among the key issues facing the workforce are:

- Insufficient workforce/treatment capacity to meet demand;
- The changing profile of those needing services (e.g., an increasing number of injecting drug users, narcotic prescription and methamphetamine users);
- A shift to increased public financing of treatment;
- Challenges related to the adoption of best practices;
- Increased utilization of medications in treatment;
- A movement toward a recovery management model of care (i.e., a chronic care approach analogous to those adopted for the treatment of other chronic disorders, such as diabetes and heart disease);
- Provision of services in generalist and specialist settings (e.g., provision of services in primary care and other settings in addition to addictions treatment program settings);

- Use of performance and patient outcome measures; and
- Discrimination associated with addictions.

Stakeholder Priority Recommendations by Focus Area

Following the context, the report includes a listing of stakeholder priority recommendations for key focus areas and a detailed discussion for each focus area and recommendation. In total, 21 stakeholder recommendations are presented in this report. These recommendations represent the most critical subset among a larger group of recommendations that stakeholders made.

A. Infrastructure Development Priorities

1. Create career paths for the treatment and recovery workforce and adopt national core competency standards;
2. Establish a National Addictions Health Professional Services Corps Loan Forgiveness and Repayment Program;
3. Foster network development; and
4. Provide technical assistance to enhance the capacity to use information technology.

B. Leadership and Management Priorities

1. Develop, deliver and sustain training for treatment and recovery support supervisors, who serve as the technology transfer agents for the latest research and best practices; and
2. Develop, deliver and sustain leadership and management development initiatives.

C. Recruitment Priorities

1. Expand recruitment of health care professionals in addictions medicine;
2. Improve student recruitment with educational institutions, focusing on under-represented groups;
3. Employ marketing strategies to attract workers to the addictions treatment field; and
4. Continue efforts to reduce the stigma associated with working in addictions treatment.

D. Addictions Education and Accreditation Priorities

1. Include training on addictions as part of education programs for primary health care and for other health and human service professions (e.g., physicians, nurses, psychologists and social workers);
2. Call for the use of national addictions core competencies as the basis of curricula;
3. Support the development and adoption of national accreditation standards for addictions education programs;
4. Encourage national and State boards for the health professions to have at least 10 percent of licensing examination questions pertain to addictions;
5. Support academic programs in Historically Black Colleges and Universities (HBCUs), Hispanic Serving Institutions, Tribal Colleges and Universities and other minority-serving institutions; and
6. Develop college and university courses in addictions-related health services research and its application; and systematically disseminate research findings to academic institutions.

E. Retention Priorities

1. Identify and disseminate best practices in staff retention; and
2. Address substance misuse and relapse within the workforce.

F. Study Priorities

1. Conduct studies that examine the relationships among level of education, type of education, training and treatment outcomes;
2. Conduct studies that examine the relationships among clinician and patient/client cultural, demographic and other characteristics and treatment outcomes; and
3. Conduct studies of clinician characteristics, training and skills that enhance therapeutic alliance.

Summary

The stakeholder priority recommendations presented in *Strengthening Professional Identity* are directed at a variety of organizations. Implementation of these recommendations will require the commitment of time and resources from each of these entities.

This report was developed with the guidance of expert stakeholders from the addictions treatment and recovery field and representatives of Federal agencies. It provides a template to guide concerted action in the area of workforce development in the addictions treatment field. The future effectiveness of the addictions treatment workforce rests on its ability to invest intelligently in its future, developing systems to address issues of recruitment, retention, and staff development. Other health care professions (e.g., nurses and physicians) have demonstrated that such efforts can prove effective. It is time that the addictions treatment field, in partnership with States and the Federal government follow that example, taking the steps necessary to address the challenges faced by the addictions treatment workforce. Only by doing this will the barriers to treatment access be addressed and the quality of care substantially improved.

INTRODUCTION

> "Like other troubled industries, addictions treatment needs financial and technical investments as well as incentives to raise quality and to attract the best personnel. Indeed...without modernization and investment, the addictions treatment system will...fail to meet the public's needs" (McLellan et al., 2003).

A Workforce in Crisis: New Opportunities for Change

Addictions treatment is facing a workforce crisis. High turnover rates, worker shortages, an aging workforce, inadequate compensation, insufficient professional development, lack of defined career paths and stigma currently challenge the field. These deficiencies have a direct impact on workers and the patients/clients under their care. Further challenging the workforce are an increasingly complex patient/client population, the demand for greater accountability in patient care, limited access to information technology and the need to rapidly incorporate scientific advances into the treatment process. The addictions treatment field is composed of workers from many different professions (e.g., counselors, physicians, nurses, social workers, psychologists, marriage and family therapists, outreach and intake workers, case managers and clergy). This diversity gives the field a rich array of perspectives and skills, but also requires complex, coordinated responses to workforce issues.

While the majority of practitioners in the addictions treatment field are counselors, the roles of all professions involved in the provision of addictions treatment are critically important.

Even as the treatment system struggles with these challenges, the foundation is solidly in place to strengthen the professional identity of the workforce. The progress in science and the emerging consensus about the need for academic accreditation and national core competencies provide opportunities for the workforce to move forward with new resolve. The field is at a pivotal point in the development of its workforce. By investing in the chief asset of the treatment system—the individuals who provide addictions treatment and recovery services—significant progress can be made to address critical workforce issues.

Workforce issues in health care have gained recent prominence on the national agenda. In 2001, for example, the Institute of Medicine (IOM) produced a landmark report, *Crossing the Quality Chasm: A New Health System for the 21st Century*, which concluded that the U.S. health care system needs fundamental change. Report recommendations included a framework and strategies for achieving substantial improvements, including six approaches to improve health care and ten rules to guide the redesign of the health care system. In 2005, the IOM report *Improving the Quality of Health Care for Mental and Substance Use Conditions* included a dedicated chapter discussing the need to increase substance use and mental health workforce capacity for quality improvement. While SAMHSA has been addressing workforce issues for more than a decade, these issues have been further elevated due to concerns regarding recruitment, diminished funding, adoption of best practices and staff retention raised by the diverse professions that comprise the workforce. This report, which was developed on behalf of the addictions treatment field, is intended to serve as a catalyst and guide for the development of national, State and local strategies that address addictions treatment workforce issues.

In 1999, prior to the IOM report, SAMHSA convened a Workforce Issues Panel as part of the National Treatment Plan Initiative to examine workforce issues related to addictions treatment. The Panel recommended (1) creating a national platform within SAMHSA to address addictions workforce issues; (2) developing and strengthening an infrastructure to attract, support and maintain a competent and diverse workforce representative of the patient/client population; and (3) improving workforce competency by providing education and training rooted in evidence-based knowledge.

In 2003, recognizing the need for more comprehensive information about the workforce, SAMHSA commissioned an environmental scan of the recent research related to the treatment workforce. The environmental scan identified five specific needs:

- Quantitative data on the workforce;
- Educational standards and workforce credentialing;
- Training to raise skill levels of the existing workforce;
- Strategies to reduce stigma; and
- Strategies to address an aging workforce (Kaplan, 2003).

Following the environmental scan, SAMHSA's Center for Substance Abuse Treatment (CSAT) convened 128 individuals representing diverse stakeholder groups in nine separate stakeholder meetings from January through May 2004. During these meetings, CSAT solicited information and recommendations from representatives knowledgeable about the exceptional challenges faced by the addictions treatment workforce. Individuals from the following organizations and employment categories provided input: Addiction Technology Transfer Centers, certification boards, Federal agencies, professional trade associations, addictions counselors, clinical supervisors, college and university professors, faith-based providers, human resource managers, marriage and family therapists, nurses, physicians, psychiatrists, recovery support personnel, researchers, social workers, State Directors and treatment providers. (See Section IV for a list of individuals who participated in these discussions.) This report includes recommendations that emerged from these expert panels.

The Addictions Treatment Workforce

The nature of the addictions treatment workforce has changed substantially over the past 30 years. Prior to the mid-1970s, recovering individuals provided counseling services with minimal formal training. In the late 1970s, States and national associations established professional standards and credentialing processes (Keller and Dermatis, 1999). Credentialing bodies now exist in every State, and a college degree is the norm rather than the exception for professionals in the field. Eighty percent of direct care treatment staff, for example, hold a bachelor's degree (Johnson et al., 2002; Knudsen et al., 2003; RMC Research Corporation, 2003) and 53 percent have a master's degree or above (Harwood, 2002).

Remarkable advances in scientific knowledge, professional development and standards of care have enabled addictions treatment to emerge as a specialty health care discipline. However, problems related to infrastructure, recruitment, retention and education and training of the workforce create an environment in which it is increasingly difficult to implement the most effective treatment. The challenges to maintaining a qualified workforce are numerous. Greater academic demands are being placed on treatment professionals. Many individuals who have traditionally entered the workforce may be discouraged from working in the field, either because of the increasing academic requirements, because compensation is inadequate to justify the investment of time and monetary resources required to obtain additional educational training, or because workloads and schedules make it difficult or impossible to complete the required academic training.

Concurrently, the Federal government has invested new resources to expand treatment. Appropriations for addictions treatment have increased from \$1.9 billion in FY 1996 to nearly \$2.8 billion in FY 2004, or by 43.9 percent over this eight-year period (ONDCP, 2004). However, relatively few resources have been dedicated to strengthening the human infrastructure that provides treatment services.

As scientific knowledge in the field of addictions treatment has expanded and the levels of credentialing have increased, one thing has remained constant: the exceptional level of passion and dedication that counselors, other professionals in the field and volunteers bring to their work. While the field currently faces a variety of challenges, the sense of mission that drives the treatment workforce gives it both a unique history and a unique resilience. Efforts to address workforce issues in the addictions treatment field need to build on this foundation and tap into the extraordinary assets that addictions professionals regularly evidence.

Rejuvenating the workforce will take a concerted effort over time. The extent of the workforce crisis is such that immediate action is required. While the issues are complex, the consequences of failing to act are enormous. By confronting the challenges head on and seizing opportunities to strengthen the workforce, we will lay the groundwork for improving quality of care.

Organization of This Report

This report consists of four sections:

- Section I: Context: Trends Impacting the Workforce
- Section II: Recommendations
    - A. Infrastructure Development Priorities
    - B. Leadership and Management Priorities
    - C. Recruitment Priorities
    - D. Addictions Education and Accreditation Priorities
    - E. Retention Priorities
    - F. Study Priorities
- Section III: Summary
- Section IV: Participants

Section I provides a historical context, discussing finance practices, demographics, and regulatory and practice trends relevant to understanding current workforce issues and the kinds of strategies that will be required to address them. This section provides a background for the recommendations that follow. Section II lists and categorizes recommendations that emerged from the stakeholder meetings. Although these categories overlap, they provide a useful framework for a systematic analysis of the recommendations. Section III provides a summary of the report. Finally, Section IV lists and acknowledges stakeholder meeting participants and other individuals who contributed to the development of the report.

References

Harwood, H.J., "Survey on Behavioral Health Workplace," *Frontlines: Linking Alcohol Services Research and Practice,* (Bethesda, MD: NIAAA, 2002).

Institute of Medicine (IOM), *Crossing the Quality Chasm: A New Health System for the 21st Century,* (Washington, DC: National Academy Press, 2001).

Johnson, J.A., H.K. Knudsen and P.M. Roman, "Counselor Turnover in Private Facilities," *Frontlines: Linking Alcohol Services Research and Practice,* (Bethesda, MD: NIAAA, 2002).

Kaplan, L., *Substance Abuse Treatment Workforce Environmental Scan,* (Washington, DC: Abt Associates Inc., 2003).
Keller, D.S. and H. Dermatis, "Current Status of Professional Training in the Addictions," *Substance Abuse* 20(3), 1999, pp. 123-140.
Knudsen, H.K., J.A. Johnson and P.M. Roman, "Retaining Counseling Staff at Substance Abuse Treatment Centers: Effects of Management Practices," *Journal of Substance Abuse Treatment* 24(2), 2003, pp. 129-135.
McLellan, A.T., D. Carise and H.D. Kleber, "Can the National Addictions Treatment Infrastructure Support the Public's Demand for Quality Care?" *Journal of Substance Abuse Treatment* 25(2), 2003, pp. 117-121.
Office of National Drug Control Policy (ONDCP), *National Drug Control Strategy: FY 2005 Budget Summary,* (Washington, DC: ONDCP, 2004).
RMC Research Corporation, "Results of a Statewide Needs Assessment of Substance Abuse Treatment Professionals," *Kentucky Workforce Survey 2002,* (Portland, OR: RMC, 2003).

I. Context: Trends Impacting the Workforce

The purpose of this section is to provide a context for understanding and addressing both longstanding and emergent workforce issues. The addictions treatment field and the social, economic and political contexts in which the workforce operates have evolved significantly over the past 30 years. While many of the challenges facing the addictions treatment workforce have remained relatively constant over time, others have emerged more recently.

Among the key issues facing the workforce are:

- Insufficient workforce/treatment capacity to meet demand;
- The changing profile of those needing services;
- A shift to increased public financing of treatment;
- Challenges related to the adoption of best practices;
- Increased utilization of medications in treatment;
- A movement toward a recovery management model of care;
- Provision of services in generalist and specialist settings;
- Use of performance and patient outcome measures; and
- Discrimination associated with addictions.

Each of these issues is discussed below.

Insufficient Workforce to Meet Treatment Demands

Nationally, addictions treatment capacity is insufficient to accommodate all those seeking services and is substantially inadequate to serve the total population in need. Capacity issues vary by geographic area, population and the type of treatment required. Per capita funding for treatment services also differs by State. Some States are able to invest substantial State and local resources into treatment, whereas others rely primarily on Federal funding. Given limited resources, States and localities are faced with difficult decisions, such as limiting the types or number of services individuals can receive and/or limiting the number of individuals who can receive services. Moreover, in recent years, many States have experienced severe revenue shortfalls that have reduced treatment capacity, despite Federal budget increases.

When treatment systems are required to provide additional services with less funding, providers and the workforce experience enormous pressures. Additionally, a large number of individuals are unable to access care due to limited workforce capacity.

The *2004 National Survey on Drug Use and Health* (NSDUH, 2005), which collected data on self-reported drug and alcohol use, found that:

> Approximately 23.48 million individuals age 12 and older needed specialty treatment for alcohol or illicit drug problems;
>
> 2.33 million of these individuals received treatment at a specialty facility;
>
> Of the 21.15 million persons who were determined to need but did not receive treatment, only 1.2 million acknowledged a need for treatment; and
>
> Of the 1.2 million persons who felt that they needed treatment, 792,000 did not attempt to access it, and 441,000 reported that they were unable to access treatment.

The high costs of not treating alcohol and drug abuse are well documented. Economic costs associated with alcohol abuse are estimated to be $184.6 billion and the costs of drug abuse are estimated to be $143 billion (Mark et al., 2005). These include the medical costs associated with alcohol and drug abuse, lost earnings linked to premature death, lost productivity, motor vehicle crashes, crime and other social consequences. The data further reflect that treating substance use disorders can result in cost benefits for many other systems, such as primary health care, child welfare, welfare and criminal justice (NIDA, 1999).

The capacity constraints that the field faces go beyond limited treatment resources. Capacity is also limited by the lack of a sufficient number of skilled practitioners. Treatment capacity at any level cannot exist without a viable workforce, and treatment organizations are currently struggling to recruit, hire, train and retain staff to respond to the demand for services. When available, increases in treatment dollars are primarily used to expand capacity to serve the greatest number of individuals, often neglecting the workforce infrastructure. Low salaries, minimal benefits, high turnover and staff dissatisfaction make recruiting staff to expand capacity a mounting challenge. (A table showing the median salary of addictions counselors and of similar professions in 2000, the most recent year for which data is available, can be found in Section II, under *Retention Issues*, below.) Additionally, the emergent issues discussed in this section are creating further pressure on an inadequately sized workforce that is battling to keep pace with these new demands. To meet these demands, the workforce will need to adopt a new way of doing business. Intensive technology transfer efforts will be required to make this possible.

The addictions treatment system has been under-funded for many years. As a result, providers often do not have the infrastructure to prioritize training, provide regular salary increases and make technology improvements, much less expand service provision and implement evidence-based practices. Because of the chronic nature of the funding crisis experienced by publicly funded treatment providers, there is a tendency to view the status quo as the norm or as an acceptable standard. The service system requires additional resources to effectively support the provision of services at current levels. Expansion of capacity will require an even more significant investment in infrastructure. Broad adoption of evidence-based practices and implementation of effective quality improvement and performance monitoring systems will require a greater investment. Investment that does not attend to infrastructure deficits is not likely to generate the quality of outcomes desired.

The Changing Profile of Those Needing Services

Over the past decade, drug use patterns and resultant treatment needs have substantively changed. For example:

- The preferred route of drug administration among youth changed from inhalation to injection from 1992 to 2000, with the rate of injection among heroin users increasing from 34 to 51 percent among those under age 18 and from 48 to 63 percent among those ages 18 to 24 (SAMHSA, 2003).

- The numbers of persons using prescription pain relievers non-medically for the first time increased from 600,000 in 1990 to more than 2 million in 2001 (NSDUH, 2004a).
- The number of older adults with substance use disorders is expected to increase from 2.5 million persons in 1999 to 5 million persons by 2020, a 100 percent increase (Gfroerer et al., 2002).

Admission patterns to treatment facilities also changed significantly from 1992 to 2002 (see Figure 1.). For instance, admissions for alcohol dependence and abuse declined from 59 percent to 42 percent, and admissions for cocaine declined from 18 percent to 13 percent. These decreases were offset, however, by increases in admissions for marijuana/hashish users from 6 percent to 15 percent, for primary opiate users from 12 percent to 18 percent and for stimulant users from 1 percent to 7 percent. Among youth 15 to 17 years of age, admissions for marijuana rose from 23 percent to 63 percent (SAMHSA, 2004b). These data point to the necessity of having a workforce prepared to respond to changes in both drug use and patient characteristics.

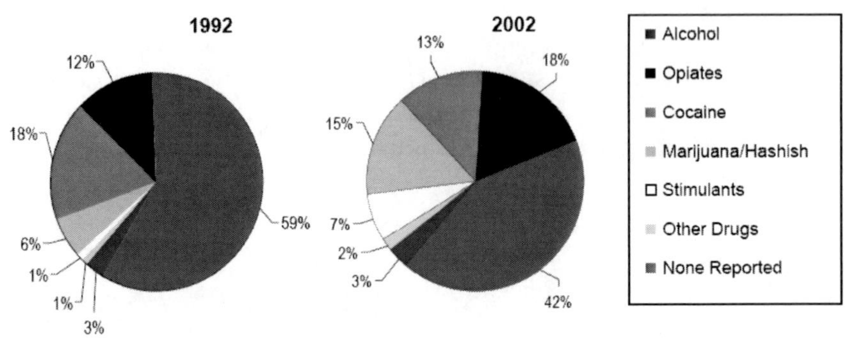

Source: SAMHSA, 2004b.

Figure 1. Primary Substance at Admission: 1992 and 2002.

The complex constellation of conditions with which individuals often present to treatment, including co-occurring mental health and substance use disorders, co-morbid medical conditions, homelessness and criminal justice or child welfare system involvement, places exceptional demands on the workforce and requires a sophisticated, multi-disciplinary approach bridging the mental health, medical and other systems.

Practitioners in generalist settings are beginning to screen for hazardous substance use patterns and potential addictive disorders. Such screening is being adopted in hospitals, emergency rooms, ambulatory clinics and other medical and non-medical settings. This practice will likely result in individuals presenting for specialty addictions services earlier in the progression of their addictive disorders. As protocols for Screening, Brief Intervention and Referral to Treatment (SBIRT) are adopted more broadly, the professionals in the addictions treatment field will increasingly be faced with two populations that, heretofore, have typically not been served. These are (1) individuals who are just beginning the progression to dependence; and (2) individuals with diagnosable dependence disorders, who are not yet ready to initiate traditional treatment but who may be willing to engage in low-demand motivational interventions that could eventually lead to treatment. Staff will need to be trained to effectively engage patients/clients in a manner that is fully cognizant of and responsive to both their clinical presentation and their readiness for change.

For many organizations, developing the capacity to more effectively treat those who are multiply impaired, those who are just beginning the progression toward dependence and those who, while dependent, are not yet ready to engage in treatment represents a significant challenge. Growing evidence indicates that the addictions treatment field must be prepared to serve populations that present with increasing levels of impairment across multiple domains, as well as populations that present earlier in the progression of a substance use disorder than in the past. Four trends related to increased severity cause concern.

- **Increased potency of illegal drugs such as marijuana and heroin.** The University of Mississippi's 2000 Marijuana Potency Monitoring Project showed that commercial grade marijuana tetrahydrocannabinol (THC) levels rose from under 2 percent in the late 1970s and early 1980s to 6.1 percent in 2000 (DEA, 2003). Also, data from the System to Retrieve Information from Drug Evidence (STRIDE) showed that the nationwide average purity for heroin from all sources measured approximately 37 percent in 2000, in contrast to 26 percent in 1991 and 7 percent in 1980 (DEA, 2001).
- **Consumption of dangerous and illegal drugs among younger users and, in particular, increased heroin addictions within this population.** The availability of high-purity heroin, which can be

snorted, has given rise to a new generation of younger users (DEA, 2001).

- **Serious medical problems among the patient/client population.** Increasingly, addictions programs are treating patients/clients with serious medical problems. According to the Centers for Disease Control and Prevention (CDC), the number of individuals living with AIDS who were exposed by injection drug use increased from 55,735 in 1998 to 68,636 in 2002, an increase of 23.1 percent (CDC, 2002a). Viral hepatitis is also a significant problem among injection drug users (IDUs). According to the CDC, 17,000 (60 percent) of the 30,000 new cases of hepatitis C in 2000 occurred among IDUs. Hepatitis B and C infections are also acquired rapidly among IDUs. Within five years of beginning drug use, 50 to 70 percent of IDUs contract hepatitis B, while 50 to 80 percent contract hepatitis C (CDC, 2002b).

  The rapid growth in methamphetamine use has led to a range of serious health problems among users. Cardiovascular problems associated with methamphetamine use include rapid heart rate, irregular heartbeat, increased blood pressure and damage to small blood vessels in the brain that can lead to stroke. Acute lead poisoning is also a growing problem among methamphetamine users, since a common method of illegal production uses lead acetate as a reagent (NIDA, 2002). Because lead poisoning in adults is associated with increased incidence of depression, aggressive behavior, antisocial behavior and brain damage, the treatment of patients/clients with lead exposure is challenging (NIDA, 2002).
- **Complex co-occurring disorders.** Complex co-occurring disorders are a significant issue among individuals in addictions treatment. According to the National Survey on Drug Use and Health (NSDUH), there were an estimated 21.4 million adults aged 18 or older with Serious Psychological Distress (SPD) in 2004. This represents 9.9 percent of all adults compared to the rate of 8.3 percent found in 2002. Among adults with SPD in 2004, 21.3 percent were dependent on or abused alcohol or illicit drugs compared to 7.9 percent of adults not experiencing SPD (SAMHSA, 2005). An even larger concern is the number of individuals entering addictions treatment with a mild or moderate mental illness.

  With respect to these individuals, the *2001-2002 National Epidemiologic Survey on Alcohol and Related Conditions* (NESARC) found that 19.7 percent of the respondents with any substance use disorder had at least one independent mood disorder during the same 12-month period. Furthermore, 17.7 percent had at least one independent anxiety disorder. Of those who sought treatment for an alcohol use disorder, 40.7 percent had at least one independent mood disorder, 33.4 percent had an independent anxiety disorder, and 33.0 percent had a drug use disorder. Moreover, among respondents with any drug use disorder who sought treatment for that disorder, 60.0 percent had at least one independent mood disorder, 42.6 percent had at least one independent anxiety disorder and 55.7 percent had a co-morbid alcohol use disorder (Grant et al., 2004). Only 9.9 percent of individuals who needed specialty addictions treatment in 2004 accessed care (NSDUH, 2005).

The NESARC provides evidence that mood and anxiety disorders must be addressed in the specialty addictions setting and that alcohol and drug use disorders must be dealt with in the generalist and specialty mental health settings. The study authors emphasize the seriousness of both substance-induced and independent mood and anxiety disorders. "Substance induced disorders," the authors point out, "have been shown to increase the risk for poor outcome of substance dependence and lifetime number of suicide attempts." Untreated, independent mood and anxiety disorders among individuals receiving addictions treatment can lead not only to relapse, but also to suicide. "Short of this ultimately adverse outcome, independent mood and anxiety disorders, particularly among individuals who have a comorbid substance use disorder, are immensely disabling" (Grant et al., 2004).

Shift to Increased Public Financing of Treatment

Individuals with substance use disorders rely on public sources of funding to a much greater extent than people with other diseases. According to *National Expenditures for Mental Health Services and Substance Abuse Treatment 1991-2001*, 76 percent of total substance use spending was from public sources, while only 45 percent of all health care was publicly financed (Mark et al., 2005). During the 10-year period covered by the report, public expenditures for substance use grew by 6.8 percent annually whereas overall public health care expenditures grew by 7.2 percent annually. Notably, private payer expenditures in the form of insurance reimbursements for substance abuse services trended in the opposite direction, falling by 1.1 percent annually while overall insurance expenditures for health care increased by 6.9 percent annually during that period. Out-of-pocket spending for addictions-related services grew by 3.2 percent annually, compared to 3.8 percent for all health (Mark et al., 2005). (See Figure 2. below.)

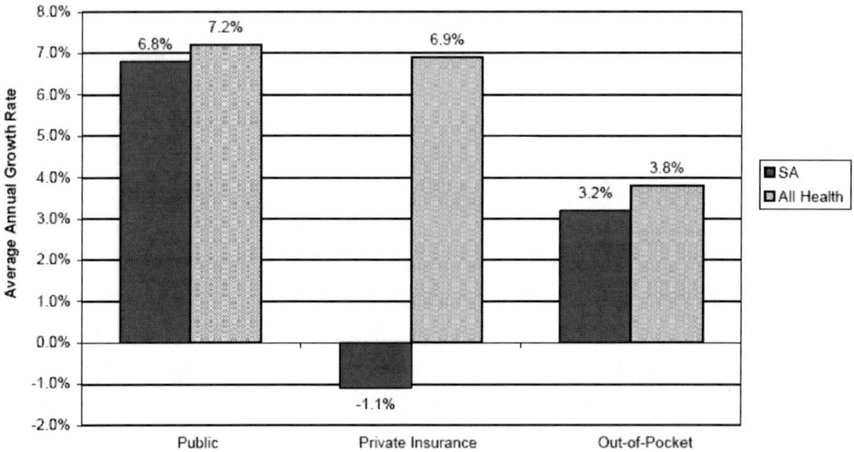

Source: Mark et al., 2005.

Figure 2. Growth of Public, Private Insurance and Out-of-Pocket Payments for Substance Abuse (SA) versus All Health, 1991-2001.

This study unequivocally points to the fact that the majority of substance use disorder treatment is financed by the public sector, that this trend is continuing and that care for substance use disorders is not financed in the same manner as other health care conditions. Though addictions impact all segments of society, lack of health coverage for treatment places enormous demands on an already overburdened publicly funded system and its workforce. Given current pressures on public funding of treatment services, particularly at the State and local levels, this decline in private insurance coverage is especially onerous.

Challenges Related to the Adoption of Best Practices

The adoption of best practices requires a stable infrastructure, organizational commitment and staff development. Indeed, the gap between what we know and what we practice is sizeable. Increasingly, the workforce is assimilating best practices into its work. Practitioners are replacing unproven approaches involving confrontation, with research-based approaches such as brief intervention, brief treatment, motivational interviewing and motivational enhancement techniques, social skills training, contingency management and community reinforcement. Many of these clinical approaches primarily focus on the use of objective feedback and empathic listening to increase a person's awareness of the potential problems caused, consequences experienced and the risks faced as a result of substance use (Rollnick and Miller, 1995).

Although the field has progressed toward incorporating best practices into its work, significant disparity remains between approaches indicated by research findings and those typically implemented by programs. Hennessy reports that the average time lag between development of an innovative practice and its adoption in practice is 17 years (Hennessy, 2004). Barriers that impede the use of evidence-based health services include resistance to change by entrenched and threatened organizational structures, outdated reimbursement rules, lack of effective provider training and lack of resources (Corrigan et al., 2001). Given these challenges related to transferring new knowledge into practice, individuals who access addictions treatment will often not receive the interventions that current research indicates are the most likely to assist them in achieving positive outcomes.

Increased Utilization of Medications in Treatment

Since the 1980s, medications for treating substance use disorders have become more available. Advances in this area have implications for improving treatment outcomes and the quality of life for patients/clients. Combining pharmacological and behavioral treatments often improves patient/client response better than either component alone. For example, just as high cholesterol can be dramatically reduced by combining diet and exercise with cholesterol-lowering medications, risk of relapse for an alcohol-dependent person can be reduced by administration of naltrexone in combination with treatment and community-based supports. Addictive disorders mirror other chronic disorders in that they often respond better to treatment approaches that extend over time, addressing physiological and neurological components of the disorder in addition to providing strategies and supports to replace unhealthy patterns with healthy ones.

Medications are used for detoxification, comorbid psychiatric conditions, opioid agonist/antagonist therapy, office-based opioid treatment, maintenance of abstinence and pain management. For example, the approval of buprenorphine by the Food and Drug Administration (FDA) provides a viable option (in addition to methadone) for addressing opiate addictions. Because it has been approved as an office-based opioid addiction treatment, buprenorphine has the potential to expand access to services by making them available in settings previously not possible, i.e., physician practices. In addition, disulfiram (antabuse) has long been used to assist individuals with alcohol dependence to abstain. Naltrexone has also been used to assist alcoholics and opiate addicts in maintaining abstinence. In July 2004, the FDA approved Campral ® (acamprosate) for assisting individuals in maintaining abstinence after withdrawing from alcohol. Acamprosate is the first medication approved for the treatment of alcoholism in a decade.

The prevalence of co-occurring mental health disorders generally requires concurrent pharmacological and psychosocial interventions, making psychotropic medications an increasingly significant component of the addictions treatment process. Moreover, the high rates of co-morbid chronic medical disorders and contagious conditions with which individuals seeking publicly funded treatment present require that programs have the ability to administer and monitor a broad array of medications, to treat conditions ranging from hypertension and high serum cholesterol to tuberculosis, hepatitis C and HIV disease.

Though attitudes are changing, some physicians remain reluctant to prescribe medications to treat addictive disorders or co-occurring mental health disorders. In addition, many treatment professionals still harbor negative perceptions about the use of pharmaceutical interventions. The increasing use of medications has the following significant workforce implications:

- Creates increased demand for nurses, physicians and other health care practitioners to prescribe, administer and monitor medication;
- Requires practitioners to learn to assess potential medication needs and to incorporate pharmacological interventions into treatment plans and treatment protocols; and
- Results in further rapprochement between the specialist treatment and generalist medical care systems to bridge workforce gaps when they cannot be filled through hiring. This could well manifest itself as co-location of generalist and specialist staff in both systems.

Over the next decade, the ability to use medications to treat both mental health and addictive disorders will become increasingly important. The demands on the workforce will be significant and cross-systems collaboration will be essential to make available the kinds of multidisciplinary teams necessary to effectively provide care in this environment. States and localities have varying requirements with respect to medical staffing in addictions treatment programs. Some require programs to have medical and nursing staff, while others have no such requirements. Moreover, there is wide variation in the level of medical staffing across programs even within jurisdictions. A recent national study found that only 54 percent of "programs had even a part-time physician on staff. Outside of methadone programs, less than 15 percent of programs employed a nurse" (McLellan et al., 2003). Mechanisms for recruiting and training additional physicians, nurses and other primary health care practitioners will need to be found.

Movement Toward a Recovery Management Model of Care

Although substance use disorders are often chronic, conventional treatment approaches have typically used acute models of care. As Dennis, Scott and Funk (2003) note:

> Longitudinal studies have repeatedly demonstrated that addictions treatment (particularly for 90 or more days) is associated with major reductions in substance use, problems and costs to society ... However, post-discharge relapse and eventual re-admission are also the norm ...The risk of relapse does not appear to abate until 4 to 5 years of abstinence ... Retrospective and prospective treatment studies report that most clients undergo 3 to 4 episodes of care before reaching a stable state of abstinence ... In spite of this evidence of chronicity and multiple episodes of care, most ... treatment continues to be characterized as relatively self-encapsulated, serial episodes of acute treatment with post discharge aftercare typically limited to passive referrals to self-help groups.

In the past 15 years, the primary health care field has developed a new approach to the treatment and management of chronic health care disorders such as diabetes mellitus, hypertension and asthma. This approach is called "disease management." Managed care organizations have built disease management protocols into requirements for the treatment of chronic conditions, such as diabetes. Segments of the addictions treatment field are beginning to evaluate how they can apply similar models. Such models are critically important as the use of medication-assisted therapies for substance use disorders becomes more prevalent, and as the profile of the publicly-funded addictions patient/client becomes more complex, involving an increasing variety of co-morbid medical and psychiatric conditions that must be managed in concert with the substance use disorder.

The disease/recovery management concept applied to addictions treatment focuses on interventions that strengthen and extend the length of remission periods, reduce the number, intensity and duration of relapse events and quickly re-engage individuals in services at the time of relapse. Recovery management models:

- Apply new advances in scientific research and practice;
- Build upon peer-to-peer support, a practice used traditionally in the field;
- Involve individuals in the management of their own illnesses;
- Implement best practices with a professionally trained workforce, supported by trained recovery specialists;
- Use case management to ensure continuity of care;
- Place greater emphasis on the long-term recovery process as opposed to a specific treatment episode; and
- Incorporate monitoring support (e.g., check-ups) throughout treatment, using the results to guide the course of subsequent care.

States are including disease/recovery management in their substance use disorder treatment services. For example, the State of Connecticut has designated the concept of "recovery" as the overarching goal of its delivery system for mental health and addictions services. Through identified model programs, it has created Centers for Excellence in key recovery-oriented areas: outreach and engagement, cultural competency, person-centered planning, peer-run programs, core skills and supported community living. The State of Arizona has revised its Medicaid plan for addictions services to include peer-delivered recovery support through the full continuum of care. Findings to date on the application of recovery management principles are encouraging. For example, a recent NIDA-funded study of individuals (n = 448) randomly assigned to recovery management checkups (RMCs), assessments, motivational interviewing and linkage to treatment re-entry, found that participants assigned to RMCs were significantly more likely than those in the control group to return to treatment, to return to treatment sooner and to spend more subsequent days in treatment. They were also significantly less likely to be in need of additional treatment at 24 months (Dennis et al., 2003).

Preliminary research indicates that recovery management approaches hold great promise. To the extent that States and treatment provider organizations adopt such approaches, the workforce will not only need training and support to integrate these protocols, but will also need to establish networks with a variety of traditional and non-traditional partners.

Provision of Services in Generalist and Specialist Settings

A diverse group of individuals within the addictions treatment workforce provides services in two sectors: the generalist and specialist treatment sectors. The generalist setting consists of primary health care centers and other community settings (e.g., trauma centers/emergency rooms, ob-gyn clinics, occupational medicine programs, schools with student assistance programs and student health services, welfare offices and work sites with employee assistance programs). The specialist setting is designed to treat individuals with substance use disorders. It consists of specialized services provided by not-for-profit, and for-profit organizations and by private practitioners. The vast majority of specialty addictions treatment is provided through community-based, not-for-profit agencies with public funds.

At present, the following activities are beginning to be implemented in selected generalist settings:

- Screening for alcohol and drug problems;
- Brief intervention and brief treatment for non-dependent users; and
- Referral and follow-up to the specialist treatment system for dependent users.

Historically, generalist staff have usually not screened and provided services related to substance use problems, and addictions treatment specialist staff have rarely been stationed in generalist settings to provide such services. However, changes are occurring due to a recognized need to intervene with individuals before high-risk behaviors progress to a diagnosable substance use disorder. Very few generalist setting staff have been trained in substance use disorders. They lack the knowledge to detect such problems. To help overcome these barriers, SAMHSA developed the SBIRT initiative. In FY 2006, this effort is being implemented in nine States. An evaluation of this $30 million effort is underway, so that the field may benefit from the knowledge gained from it.

The diversity of the population with substance use problems requires the workforce to be equipped to address issues as they arise in both the generalist and specialist settings. A large segment of the population would benefit greatly from earlier detection of this illness, potentially reducing the number of individuals who would eventually require specialty treatment. However, the workforce within the generalist setting is not prepared to address this issue in a significant manner without substantially more education and training.

The complexity of the specialist setting raises unique challenges for workforce development across both the public and private sectors. Not only do funding mechanisms and minimum staffing and care requirements vary greatly from State to State, but publicly and privately funded organizations have differing priorities, incentives, organizational cultures, philosophies, service mixes and target populations. Additionally, the workforce within the specialist setting has ongoing training needs due to changing treatment technology, staff turnover and recent initiatives to begin engaging individuals in the early stages of substance use problems through co-location or linkage with generalist settings. Cross-training of generalists and specialists is critically important. The magnitude of this disease and the scarcity of resources dedicated to its treatment require that the two settings work together to meet the challenges that drug and alcohol use present.

Use of Performance and Patient Outcome Measures

The addictions field is experiencing increasing demands for accountability in treatment performance. Funding entities and service providers want quantitative feedback on the benefits experienced by service recipients and on measures necessary for enhanced treatment efficiency and effectiveness. The Washington Circle Group, "a multi-disciplinary group of providers, researchers, managed care representatives and public policy makers" convened by SAMHSA in 1998 to develop a core set of performance measures for addictions treatment, has noted that "monitoring the quality and availability of alcohol and other drug services must be a central tenet of any health-related performance measurement system." The Washington Circle Group has further noted that "performance measures for alcohol and other drugs need to become an integral part of a comprehensive set of behavioral and physical health performance measures for managed care plans" (Washington Circle Group, 2005).

SAMHSA has required the collection of National Outcome Measures (NOMs) to track outcomes and performance related to treatment services funded under the Substance Abuse Prevention and Treatment Block Grant. All States are required to report by September 2007. Discretionary grantees are already reporting NOMs. NOMs will track outcomes and performance across 10 domains: 1) abstinence; 2) employment/education; 3) crime and criminal justice; 4) housing stability; 5) access/capacity; 6) retention; 7) social connectedness; 8) perception of care; 9) cost-effectiveness; and 10) use of evidence-based practices. To support States in their data collection and reporting, SAMHSA will provide infrastructure and technical assistance through a new State Outcomes Measurement and Management System (SOMMS). Because the majority of addictions treatment services nationally are publicly funded, NOMs will become one of the most broadly adopted sets of outcomes/performance measures.

Nationally, across both private and public sector managed care plans, the Health Plan Employer Data and Information Set (HEDIS) is the most widely adopted package of performance measures (Washington Circle Group, 2004). Developed by the National Committee for Quality Assurance (NCQA), HEDIS is a set of standardized performance measures designed to permit reliable comparison of the performance of managed health care plans (NCQA, 2005). Until 2003, it included no performance measures related to the treatment of addictive disorders.

In February 2003, NCQA added two measures specific to substance use disorders that had been developed by the Washington Circle Group: 1) *Identification of Alcohol and Other Drug Services*, which tracks the percentage of plan members who initiate addictions treatment services and the type of service provided; and 2) *Initiation and Engagement of Alcohol and Other Drug Dependence Treatment*, which measures the percentage of plan members who receive two or more additional substance use disorder services within 30 days of initiation (NCQA, 2003).

In a report entitled *Rewarding Results: Improving the Quality of Treatment for People with Alcohol and Drug Problems,* a national policy panel headed by Jerome Jaffe, M.D., affirmed the Washington Circle Group's performance measures. However, the panel recognized that a "weak infrastructure dramatically limits the effectiveness of many basic quality improvement strategies." The panel acknowledged that "many programs are well run and provide high quality care," but pointed out that "too many are fiscally weak and unstable." The panel argued that "only in a more stable treatment system can we hope to use training to achieve significant increments in quality" (Join Together, 2003).

To begin developing a stable infrastructure upon which to build training, technology transfer and quality improvement systems, the panel report recommended that public and private funders financially reward programs with good results, such as reduced drug and alcohol use, reduced medical services utilization, reduced criminal justice system involvement and increased employment. Acknowledging the difficult truth that doing so would mean "taking patients and funds from programs with consistently poor results," the panel recognized that weaker programs would likely need to close or consolidate with other programs. However, the panel expected that under such financial incentives, "new partnerships should evolve among providers that help them preserve their viability without total merger – for example, arrangements that allow them to share specialized personnel and administrative or technology costs" (Join Together, 2003).

Systems that provide financial incentives for the provision of quality care offer hope for the field, but also represent a significant challenge for provider organizations and clinicians and may be perceived by many organizations and professionals as more of a threat than an opportunity. However, it will require committed efforts of this kind on the national, State and local levels to significantly improve the quality of addictions treatment. Such efforts would go a long way toward securing for the field the recognition and central role in health care systems that it merits. The field must play such a role to effectively address the addictions treatment needs faced within the United States.

Discrimination Associated with Addictions and the Addictions Treatment Workforce

Negative perceptions of addictions have far-reaching results that go beyond their impact on the treatment workforce. A Join Together issue paper says rampant discrimination restricts access to education, housing, employment, financial assistance and health care for people with addictions (2001). Some examples are:

- Insurance policies that deny or restrict coverage for addictions treatment;

- The Drug Free Student Aid provision of the U.S. Higher Education Act, which denies financial aid to students with a drug conviction; and
- The 1996 welfare reform provision that imposes a lifetime ban on welfare benefits for people convicted of possessing or selling drugs.

According to *The Christian Science Monitor*, experts in treatment and recovery estimate that when recovering individuals are honest about their drug histories, they will be turned down for a job 75 percent of the time (Marks, 2002). A Join Together feature article cites a California survey in which 59 percent of employers said they would never hire anyone with a felony conviction (Curley, 2002).

As noted above, discrimination also results in avoidance of treatment, often delaying care until the substance use disorder has progressed substantially and/or complex co-occurring disorders emerge or worsen. Among one million people who were identified as needing treatment and who felt that they needed it, but did not receive it, 19.6 percent reported that they did not try to access it due to the stigma associated with addictions (NSDUH, 2004b). The net result of such treatment avoidance is that individuals present to treatment later with more complicated needs. They are subsequently more costly to treat than they would have been had an intervention occurred earlier. Effectively addressing stigma around addictions could result in more timely intervention, improved outcomes and reduced health care costs.

Discrimination also affects the addictions treatment professional. Many believe that the stigma attached to addictions results in decreased funding to address workforce issues and has a detrimental effect on attracting and retaining professionals in the workforce. Addictions treatment struggles to be recognized as a field that provides vital health care for a life-threatening chronic disorder.

Implications of Current Trends

Over the past decade, trends have reflected the increasing pressures experienced by the addictions treatment workforce. Individuals entering treatment are presenting with more complex and severe disorders while resources have remained relatively scarce. Private health plan coverage of addictions treatment has declined in fixed dollars and as a percentage of overall health plan coverage over the past decade, placing even greater demands on a system that was already inadequately funded to meet demand. In

1991, private insurance accounted for 24 percent of substance abuse treatment expenditures, whereas, in 2001, it accounted for only 13 percent (Mark et al., 2005). At the same time, the profile of the publicly funded addictions treatment patient/client has changed. Clinicians and programs must be prepared to address the needs of both a more severely impaired population, with problems that are more numerous and more intractable, and a less impaired population that is being referred earlier in the progression of an addictive disorder. To maintain skills that will keep pace with the rapidly changing environment, the workforce must be resilient, clinically competent and adaptable. Addressing these challenges will require ongoing knowledge and skill development at the executive, management and practitioner levels, and will also require diversification of the workforce through specialization among counselors and through the addition of a larger number of allied professionals. Specialized expertise is needed in areas such as brief treatment, medication-assisted therapies and co-occurring disorders.

References

Centers for Disease Control and Prevention (CDC), *HIV/AIDS Surveillance Report: Cases of HIV and AIDS in the United States, 2002*, (Atlanta, GA: CDC, 2002a).

Centers for Disease Control and Prevention (CDC), *Viral Hepatitis and Injection Drug Users*, (Atlanta, GA: CDC, 2002b).

Corrigan, P.W., L. Steiner, S.G. McCracken, B. Blaser and M. Barr, "Strategies for Disseminating Evidence-based Practices to Staff Who Treat People With Serious Mental Illness," *Psychiatric Services* 52(12), 2001, pp. 1598-1606.

Curley, B., "Discrimination Against People in Recovery Rampant, Advocates Say," *Join Together Online*, 2002, *Online*, <http://www.jointogether.org/sa/news/features/reader/0,1854,553416,00.html>, Oct. 2004.

Dennis, M., C.K. Scott and R. Funk, "An Experimental Evaluation of Recovery Management Checkups (RMC) for People with Chronic Substance Use Disorders," *Evaluation and Program Planning* 26(3), 2003, pp. 339-352.

Drug Enforcement Administration (DEA), *Illegal Drug Price and Purity Report*, (Washington, DC: DEA, 2003).

Drug Enforcement Administration (DEA), "Drug Trafficking in the United States," (Washington, DC: DEA, 2001), *Online*, <www.dea.gov /concern /drug trafficking.html>, Oct. 2004.

Gfroerer, J.C., M.A. Penne, M.R. Pemberton and R.E. Folsom, "The Aging Baby Boom Cohort and Future Prevalence of Substance Abuse," *Substance Use by Older Adults: Estimates of Future Impact on the Treatment System*, (Rockville, MD: DHHS, SAMHSA, 2002).

Grant, B.F., F.S. Stinson, D.A. Dawson, S.P. Chou, M.C. Dufour, W. Compton, R.P. Pickering and K. Kaplan, "Prevalence and Co-occurrence of Substance Use Disorders and Independent Mood and Anxiety Disorders: Results From the National Epidemiologic Survey on Alcohol and Related Conditions," *Archives of General Psychiatry* 61(8), 2004, pp. 807-816.

Hennessy, K.D., *SAMHSA's Science to Services Initiative and Expansion of the National Registry of Effective Practices and Programs (NREPP)*, Presentation to 14th Anniversary Conference on SMHA Services Research, Program Evaluation and Policy, 2004, *Online*, <http://www.nri-inc.org/Conference/Conf04/Presentations/Hennessy.pdf>, Jan. 2005.

Join Together Online, "Hot Issues: Discrimination," 2001, *Online*, <http://www.jointogether.org/sa/issues/hot issues/discrimination/more/>, Oct. 2004.

Join Together Online, "Rewarding Results: Improving the Quality of Treatment for People with Alcohol and Drug Problems: Recommendations from a National Policy Panel," 2003, *Online*, <http://www.jointogether.org/sa/files/pdf/quality.pdf>, March 2005.

Mark, T., R.M. Coffey, D. McKusick, H. Harwood, E. King, E. Bouchery, J. Genuardi, R. Vandivort, J.A. Buck and J. Dilonardo, *National Expenditures for Mental Health Services and Substance Abuse Treatment, 1991-2000*, (Rockville, MD: DHHS, SAMHSA, 2005).

Marks, A., "Jobs Elude Former Drug Addicts," *The Christian Science Monitor*, 2002, *Online*, <http://www.csmonitor.com/2002/0604/p02s02-ussc.html>, Oct. 2004.

McLellan, A.T., D. Carise and H. Kleber, "Can the National Addictions Treatment Infrastructure Support the Public's Demand for Quality Care?" *Journal of Substance Abuse Treatment* 25(2), 2003, pp. 117-121.

National Committee for Quality Assurance (NCQA), "NCQA Releases HEDIS 2004, 10 New Measures Address Public Health, Service Issues," 2003, *Online,* <http://www.ncqa.org/communications/news/hedis2004. htm>, March 2005.

National Committee for Quality Assurance (NCQA), "What is HEDIS?" 2005, *Online,* <http://www.ncqa.org/Programs/HEDIS/>, March 2005.

National Institute on Drug Abuse (NIDA), *NIDA Research Report – Methamphetamine Abuse and Addictions*, (Rockville, MD: NIH, 2002).

National Institute on Drug Abuse (NIDA), *Principles of Drug Addictions Treatment: A Research Based Guide,* (Rockville, MD: NIH, 1999), *Online*, <http://www.drugabuse.gov/PDF/PODAT/PODAT.pdf>, Oct. 2004.

National Survey on Drug Use and Health (NSDUH), "Nonmedical Use of Prescription Pain Relievers," *The NSDUH Report,* (Rockville, MD: SAMHSA, 2004a), *Online*, <http://oas.samhsa.gov/2k4/pain/pain.htm>, Oct. 2004.

National Survey on Drug Use and Health (NSDUH), *Results from the 2003 National Survey on Drug Use and Health: National Findings,* (Rockville, MD: SAMHSA, 2004b), *Online,* <http://www.oas.samhsa.gov/nhsda/2k3 nsduh/2k3Results.htm>, March 2005.

Rollnick, S. and W.R. Miller, "What is Motivational Interviewing?" *Behavioral and Cognitive Psychotherapy*, Vol. 23, 1995, pp. 325-334, *Online*, <http://www.motivationalinterview.org/clinical/whatismi.html>, Oct. 2004.

Substance Abuse and Mental Health Services Administration (SAMHSA), *The DASIS Report: New Heroin Users Admitted to Substance Abuse Treatment: 1992-2000,* (Rockville, MD: OAS, 2003), *Online*, <http://oas.samhsa.gov/2k3/newHeroinTX/newHeroinTX.cfm>, Oct. 2004.

Substance Abuse and Mental Health Services Administration (SAMHSA), *Overview of Findings from the 2003 National Survey on Drug Use and Health,* (Rockville, MD: DHHS, 2004a).

Substance Abuse and Mental Health Services Administration (SAMHSA), *Treatment Episode Data Set (TEDS) Highlights—2002. National Admissions to Substance Abuse Treatment Services,* (Rockville, MD: DHHS, 2004b), *Online,* < http://wwwdasis.samhsa.gov/teds02/2002 teds highlights.pdf >, March 2005.

The Washington Circle Group, "Background of the WC," 2005, *Online*, <http://www.washingtoncircle.org>, March 2005.

The Washington Circle Group, "Specification of Performance Measures for the Identification, Initiation and Engagement of Alcohol and Other Drug Services," (Washington, DC: The Washington Circle, 2004), Online,

<http://www.washingtoncircle.org/Final%20Specs%202004_03-30.pdf>, March 2005.

II. RECOMMENDATIONS

The Recommendations section summarizes the input from the diverse stakeholders, cites relevant literature and makes recommendations across major topic areas including the identity of the addictions treatment field and the challenges and opportunities it faces. It is intended to guide the development of organizational, local, State and national strategies for addressing the many workforce challenges facing the addictions treatment field.

A. Infrastructure Development Priorities

Infrastructure Issues in Brief

A sound addictions treatment infrastructure ensures the availability of a qualified workforce capable of meeting the treatment and recovery needs of diverse populations. This infrastructure must include mechanisms to attract, educate, train and retain staff and to support the dynamic capacity of the treatment delivery system. The infrastructure also must include information systems that support and enhance workers' abilities to manage treatment services and ensure accountability and quality of care.

Current data indicate that more than 67,000 practitioners provide addictions treatment and related services (Harwood, 2002). By 2010, the need for addictions professionals and licensed treatment staff with graduate-level degrees is expected to increase by 35 percent (NASADAD, 2003). With anecdotal evidence already indicating a shortage of staff, more severe staffing shortages are anticipated in the near future. Exacerbating this issue is the current unmet need for treatment services. Staff workloads are high, salaries are low and employee benefits are minimal. The effects on the workforce are dramatic: staff turnover rates of nearly 20 percent and high levels of worker dissatisfaction (Knudsen et al., 2003; Gallon et al., 2003).

With treatment organizations struggling to recruit and retain staff, attracting individuals to the field to expand capacity is a challenge. A modest 10 percent increase in treatment capacity would require an additional 6,800 clinicians above the annual number currently required to replace staff leaving clinical practice (The Lewin Group, 2004). The treatment system's capacity to close the gap in alcohol and drug treatment is threatened by a lack of national occupational standards, inadequate incentives to enter the addictions treatment workforce and an absence of defined career paths.

Recommendations

To strengthen the addictions treatment infrastructure, stakeholders made the following recommendations:

1. Create career paths for the treatment and recovery workforce and adopt national core competency standards;
2. Establish a National Addictions Health Professional Services Corps Loan Forgiveness and Repayment Program;
3. Foster network development; and
4. Provide technical assistance to enhance the capacity to use information technology.

1. Create Career Paths for the Treatment and Recovery Workforce and Adopt National Core Competency Standards

Competency standards articulate expectations of professional practice and ensure that individuals holding a specific type of position have the same basic core knowledge, skill and/or ability. SAMHSA, through a consensus process, developed *Technical Assistance Publication 21* (TAP 21) *Addiction Counseling Competencies: The Knowledge, Skills and Attitudes of Professional Practice*, which defines competencies and serves as a basis for the field to move forward on national competency standards. Unfortunately, these standards have not been universally adopted. SAMHSA recently revised TAP 21 to reflect the latest science. The revised version of TAP 21 should be adopted nationally. By developing and implementing national core competency standards, variation in clinical practice will be lessened and quality of care will be improved. The Institute of Medicine's (IOM's) report, *Health Professions Education: A Bridge to Quality,* calls for the adoption of core competencies across all health professions (2003). Further, creating career paths that incorporate core competencies provides credibility to the field, and professional development and advancement opportunities for those wishing to enter the workforce.

Discussion

> "A competency is a measurable human capability that is required for effective performance. A competency may be comprised of knowledge, a single skill or ability, a personal characteristic, or a cluster of two or more of these. Competencies are the building blocks of work performance. The performance of most tasks requires the simultaneous or sequenced demonstration of multiple competencies" (Marrelli et al., 2004).

Although the addictions treatment field is relatively young, it has distinguished itself as a specialty. As in other health care fields, specialization creates the need to define standards of care and the core competencies required to provide care. While every State has a credentialing process and most States have an entry-level counselor credential (NASADAD, 2003), credentialing standards differ among States and, within a few States, there is more than one credentialing organization. In addition, there are no uniformly adopted credentialing standards for social workers, psychologists, nurses, physicians and other professionals who practice in the addictions treatment and recovery field. National core competency standards for addictions treatment professionals have not been adopted.

To garner greater legitimacy and recognition as part of mainstream health care, it is critically important that the field move forward as a discipline and adopt national competencies. It is recommended that SAMHSA/CSAT establish a collaborative process with the States and national credentialing boards to implement and periodically update national core competency standards for counselors. By adopting national core competencies, States can develop career paths incorporating practice standards recognized by the field. It is also recommended that SAMHSA/CSAT initiate dialogue with stakeholders to adopt and periodically update core competencies for other practitioners providing addictions treatment and recovery support services.

Career paths provide structure for organizations and individuals in the workforce and identify potential opportunities for career advancement. Additionally, career paths help individuals understand that they are part of a profession, validating not only training and academic credentials, but also time in the field and prior experience. For example, personal experience in recovery provides many clinicians with a unique and valuable experiential base and perspective. Moreover, many patients/clients prefer to be counseled by someone who has gone through treatment and the recovery process (McCarty, 2002). Career paths provide a mechanism for recognizing the value of this experience in addition to academic training through the range of positions that are offered on "the path."

Career paths also support the retention of competent professionals, help to identify the range of managerial, supervisory and other professional options available to those entering the field, enable workers to plan their own professional development and set career goals and give recognition and status to individuals progressing along a track to higher-level positions. As an example, a career path for an addictions counselor might begin with an entry-level position that does not require certification, licensure, degrees or extensive training and prior experience; then move to a position that requires completing a requisite number of hours of supervised clinical experience and passing a certification and/or licensure examination; and then move to an advanced level of certification or licensure that may require an advanced degree and/or additional supervised experience, and/or passing an advanced test. Such a career path could also include certification or registration in specific sub-specialties, such as treatment of adolescents or of individuals with co-occurring disorders. This career path, of course, need not end with clinical practice. It could also include program or agency management. Additional career paths will become available as the field relies more on recovery support services. By developing career paths with associated core competencies, the addictions treatment field will demonstrate its commitment to maintaining professional standards for all individuals in the treatment and recovery workforce. It is recommended that SAMHSA/CSAT convene expert stakeholders and facilitate a process leading to the development of model career paths that can serve as guidelines for State and local efforts.

The process of developing and adopting both competency standards and career paths must include evaluating current State competency and credentialing requirements and reviewing the literature related to competency modeling. In addition, the process must include coordination with certification, licensing and accreditation boards to ensure linkages and internal consistencies among all oversight bodies, and inclusion of competencies in credentialing and licensing examinations of all professionals working in the addictions treatment field (IOM, 2003). Recognizing the urgent need to act in these areas, the leadership of The Association for Addiction Professionals (NAADAC), the National Certification Commission (NCC), the International Certification and Reciprocity Consortium (IC&RC) and the Society of Credentialed Addictions Professionals (S.CAP) met in February 2005 and agreed to collaborate to advance the addictions treatment field. A proposal to consolidate existing credentials and to merge the IC&RC and NAADAC credentialing boards into a single board was submitted to the directors of the IC&RC in April 2005 and to the NAADAC leadership in July 2005.

2. Establish a National Addictions Health Professional Services Corps Loan Forgiveness and Repayment Program

A National Addictions Health Professional Services Corps Loan Forgiveness and Repayment Program, hereafter referred to as "the loan forgiveness and repayment program," would attract young and second-career professionals to the field and retain committed addictions treatment staff who seek training for professional development and recertification. Loan forgiveness and repayment programs would provide needed financial support to potential addictions professionals when low salaries make it difficult to pay for academic training. Since the 1980s and as recently as 2002, Congress has authorized loan repayment programs for teachers and some health care providers (e.g., primary care physicians, nurses). These programs have been successful in attracting and retaining individuals in professions experiencing critical staff shortages.

Discussion

A loan forgiveness and repayment program could be modeled after the National Health Services Corps (NHSC) for primary care providers. Such a program for addictions professionals would provide assistance in repayment of student loans for graduates agreeing to serve for a set period of years in communities with a critical workforce shortage. Student loan forgiveness and repayment programs are designed to encourage students to pursue academic training that will lead to employment in specific occupations. These programs forgive all or part of students' debts in exchange for working in underserved or economically disadvantaged communities.

Because of the workforce shortage in most communities nationwide, it is recommended that a loan forgiveness and repayment program for addictions professionals be made available to individuals who make a commitment to work in any community, with special consideration to those choosing to work in economically disadvantaged areas. A loan forgiveness and repayment program for addictions treatment supports the belief that individuals in the treatment workforce are a national resource and acknowledges the workforce shortage as a national crisis. A corps would provide meaningful financial incentives to physicians, nurses, social workers, psychologists, counselors and recovery support specialists who consider careers within the addictions treatment field.

The NHSC has been funded by the U.S. Department of Health and Human Services (DHHS) for 30 years and is housed in the Health Resources and Services Administration's (HRSA's) Bureau of Health Professions. It is a competitive program that makes contract awards to clinicians who agree to serve full-time at approved sites in designated health professional shortage areas for a minimum of two years. In return, NHSC participants receive funds to repay government and commercial loans for education expenses incurred during their undergraduate and health professions graduate education (DHHS/HRSA, 2004).

Since its inception, over 22,000 clinicians have participated in the NHSC nationwide. Highlights of the program's success include:

- Approximately 97 percent of clinicians fulfill their commitment;
- Approximately 60 percent of NHSC participants continue to serve their target population four years after completion of their service obligation and 52 percent continue to serve 15 years after completion of their service obligation;
- Approximately 53 percent of NHSC clinicians are from underserved populations, which is 35 percent higher than the national workforce; and
- NHSC clinicians are in every State, the District of Columbia, Puerto Rico and the Pacific Basin (Fox, 2001).

Loan forgiveness and repayment programs have demonstrated a measurable impact on recruiting and retaining clinical professionals in many communities. A 1997 GAO study of a Federal loan repayment program for physicians found that the program had a "greater impact than scholarship programs in achieving ... the objective of providing underserved communities with clinicians...and recruiting individuals motivated by a more altruistic desire to practice in underserved communities, a factor that can improve long-term retention" (DHHS/HRSA, 2004).

A national addictions loan forgiveness and repayment program is a promising idea that can increase the long-term supply of professionals in a wide range of geographic locations, and also assist with the recruitment of underrepresented groups, increasing racial, ethnic and gender diversity. Like the NHSC, a loan forgiveness and repayment program should establish partnerships with State loan repayment programs to strengthen the incentive. Further, it is recommended that components of the addictions services corps include continuing education, training and job placement assistance for individuals who complete their service obligation.

HRSA, in consultation with SAMHSA/CSAT, should develop and administer the loan forgiveness and repayment program.

3. Foster Network Development

As the field faces agency closures, particularly among smaller treatment providers, networks represent an important mechanism for ensuring agency viability and service availability. In addition, in some cases, networks can provide career paths for addictions professionals and potential staffing pools for member organizations.

Discussion

A study of the national addictions treatment infrastructure found that the organizational and administrative infrastructures of many addictions programs were inadequate and unstable (McLellan et al., 2003). In fact, of the 175 drug and alcohol treatment programs included in the study, 15 percent had either closed or stopped providing addictions treatment services. Additionally, 29 percent had been taken over or "reorganized" under a different administrative structure. In an effort to help strengthen management efficiency and ensure long-term sustainability, small addictions treatment providers may benefit from engagement in a network or use of a shared management organization to support human resource, clinical and administrative functions.

Networks can enhance the infrastructures of member agencies by making available specialized staff. For example, nursing, vocational, psychiatric, psychological, clinical social work and other services can be shared through co-location, joint funding, referral, or rotation. This sharing of resources results in economies of scale for participating agencies and also makes available critically needed supports, many of which would not be affordable otherwise to member agencies. As systems move toward evidence-based practices and expand the use of medications in treatment, affordable access to an array of specialized and relatively expensive staff resources becomes increasingly important.

In addition, networks can reduce pressure on the workforce by making available more appropriate program options and a greater pool of medical and clinical expertise than would otherwise be available. As noted above, network membership has the potential to be of particular value to smaller agencies because the resources that can be accessed (e.g., nursing and psychiatric services, shared information technology, billing, payroll and other administrative functions) enable them to function in a more cost-effective manner. The cost structures of small agencies often make operations difficult in times of economic constraint, and networking may enable them to successfully navigate periods of economic retrenchment.

To the extent that networks are formalized (e.g., via contract with each other or with a shared management organization), they can also offer viable career paths for staff working at member agencies. The operation of such a program across agencies requires a workforce development plan that is shared across network agencies and that is designed to let all network members accrue the long-term benefits of a readily accessible pool of potential employees and a more stable workforce.

When organizations join together in networks, they benefit from the ability to manage care efficiently across agencies and those they serve benefit from access to a more complete array of services. This networking has the potential to simultaneously improve efficiency of patient/client flow and cost-effectiveness. Participation in a network may also make it easier for organizations to reach their target populations and to maximize positive outcomes through an improved match between programs and patients/clients. A study has shown that when programs offer a full continuum of services, they will have the ability to better match patients/clients to services, and clinicians will have a greater sense of job satisfaction (Kauffman and Woody, 1995). It is recommended that provider organizations explore the potential benefits and feasibility of establishing formal networks.

4. Provide Technical Assistance to Enhance the Capacity to Use Information Technology

Widely available technologies to support clinical and administrative services could alleviate many workforce challenges if they were broadly adopted by the addictions treatment field. However, these technologies are cost-prohibitive for many addictions treatment agencies. The current health care environment demands that technology in the addictions treatment field be greatly improved. Technology permits clinicians, supervisors and administrators to benefit from immediate feedback and reporting to support care management, quality improvement, clinical supervision and outcomes monitoring. Greater access to information technology also provides professional development opportunities for managers and staff who want to obtain certifications and continuing education credits through the use of online training programs or Web-based university and college courses.

Discussion

Many treatment organizations lag behind their counterparts in the health care industry with regard to the ability to access and use information technology. Some small agencies do not have basic computer capabilities, much less a network, automated billing, or clinical records/clinical management systems.

Technology offers at least three important service opportunities for patients/clients and staff: (1) management of clinical practices and administrative paperwork; (2) staff participation in online learning; and (3) provider on-line patient counseling, i.e., e-therapy. The ability of providers to access and use computer technology effectively can mean the difference between whether some people—especially patients in rural areas, the physically disabled and other underserved populations—receive treatment or not (New Freedom Commission, 2003). Many people entering the field find inadequate technology in the work setting. A recent study, for example, found that 20 percent of 175 counseling centers surveyed had no information systems, e-mail or even voice-mail (McLellan et al., 2003). Further, although 50 percent of the treatment programs studied had a computerized information system available to administrative staff, these systems did not support the provision or monitoring of care. The systems were, instead, dedicated exclusively to billing or administrative record keeping.

In testimony before the National Committee on Vital Health Statistics, Thomas McLellan, Ph.D., stated that "the clinical monitoring approaches used in the treatment of other chronic illnesses are also appropriate in the treatment of addictions. These approaches stress patient responsibility for disease and lifestyle management and the early detection of relapse [and] require modern information management techniques and systems that provide standardized, relevant monitoring information to the clinician and to the payers." He further noted that "less than 40% of addictions treatment programs have information systems available for clinical decision support and clinical record keeping. This infrastructure problem is due in some part to chronically poor funding levels but even more to the fact that so many of these programs are not connected professionally, financially or clinically with the rest of mainstream health care." Recognition as a part of mainstream health care and better integration with it could go a long way in reducing the digital divide that currently separates addictions treatment from the rest of health care (McLellan, 2005).

Computer systems and the capacity to access and use modern information technology are important not only for improving administrative functions and business operations, but also for enhancing treatment services and improving the work environment. A major concern frequently expressed by clinicians is the burden of redundant paperwork (OASAS, 2002). Technology can provide effective tools to reduce the administrative workload on staff and allow more time for clinician care. "Creating, handling, filing and copying paper documents, forms and messages invariably involves more steps and time than performing the same functions electronically" (Adler, 2005). Greater efficiencies in patient/client care decrease staff workloads and improve the work environment. At the same time, recent privacy rules and guidelines on use of patient records (e.g., the Health Insurance Portability and Accountability Act [HIPAA]) may require increased use of information technology in treatment settings. Technical assistance can help treatment organizations learn about these new rules and make the best use of information technology for communication, case management, staff development and delivery of quality, patient-centered care. Funding to cover the initial cost of automating processes remains a challenge for many organizations.

Recruitment, retention and development of the addictions treatment workforce are facilitated by the availability of information technology, most especially among young adults who typically rely on computers and other technologies for accomplishing basic tasks. For those less adept with information technology, basic computer training, software and Internet access provide tools to improve clinical processes, resulting in more efficient patient/client care and information.

To assist States with technology and to support the collection, analysis and reporting of National Outcome Measures, SAMHSA has established the State Outcomes Measurement and Management System (SOMMS). Through this new system, SAMHSA, in partnership with the States, will: (1) standardize operational definitions and outcome measures; (2) link records to permit comparison of admission and discharge or post-discharge data; (3) develop benchmarking strategies to determine acceptable outcomes thresholds; and (4) produce routine management reports to direct technical assistance and the SAMHSA science-to-services program in a manner that will result in improved outcomes.

With the aid of other Operating Divisions of DHHS, it is recommended that SAMHSA develop a comprehensive information technology strategy to support States and provider organizations.

B. Leadership and Management Priorities

Leadership and Management Issues in Brief

The addictions treatment field has undergone significant changes in recent years, including a greater emphasis on accountability, patient-centered care and best practices. These changes place significant demands on the workforce, particularly leaders and managers in the field who have primary responsibility for ensuring that organizations have systems in place to support and manage the achievement of positive treatment outcomes.

The extent of the leadership and management issues in the addictions treatment field is evidenced by a 53 percent turnover rate in 2002 for program managers and directors (McLellan et al., 2003). The aging of program managers further compounds the need to develop a new generation of leaders.

Greater use of best practices has also placed new demands on staff supervisors and managers who need the knowledge and skills to reinforce new practices. Management must also provide detailed expectations of supervisors' roles and responsibilities as technology transfer agents to make the adoption of evidence-based practices successful (Heathfield, 2004).

Training alone is not adequate to ensure full and effective application of practices and their sustainability over time. In cases where practice differs from past methods, intensive supervision is essential to ensure that technology transfer occurs. As noted in *The Change Book*, "too often brief flurries of training alone are thought to be sufficient in bringing about lasting change. The results are usually short-lived alterations in practice followed by discouragement and a return to familiar but less effective ways of doing things" (ATTC, 2004). A technology transfer strategy is required to ensure effective adoption of evidence-based best practices. Technology transfer "involves creating a mechanism by which a desired change is accepted, incorporated and reinforced at all levels of an organization or system" (ATTC, 2004). For best practices to be adopted, leadership and management must develop a technology transfer strategy to ensure long-lasting organizational change.

Recommendations

To address these workforce development issues, stakeholders made the following recommendations:

1. Develop, deliver and sustain training for treatment and recovery support supervisors, who serve as the technology transfer agents for the latest research and best practices; and
2. Develop, deliver and sustain leadership and management development initiatives.

1. Develop, Deliver and Sustain Training for Treatment and Recovery Support Supervisors, Who Serve As the Technology Transfer Agents for the Latest Research and Best Practices

Clinical supervisors are critical in sustaining and developing staff competencies and must become a key focus of professional development efforts. Further, training for clinical supervisors must be based on a set of core competencies. Given the increased attention being placed on patient/client outcomes, the role of clinical supervisors as technology transfer agents is vital. Training specifically targeting recovery support services supervisors is also necessary.

Discussion

Clinical supervisors serve a number of functions in treatment organizations. They function as clinical skill developers, technology transfer agents and role models who influence retention of new and experienced staff (Culbreth, 1999; NAADAC, 2003). Because clinical supervision is not a reimbursable activity in most States, many supervisors carry caseloads in addition to their administrative and managerial responsibilities. Clinical supervision provides support for practitioners struggling with the day-to-day pressures of the job and enhances clinical skills and professional growth. Effective supervision, by monitoring the delivery of treatment services, serves as part of the quality improvement process. Simply stated, clinical supervision is sound management practice.

Scientific advances and the emphasis on patient/client outcomes have heightened the need for well-trained, highly skilled and dedicated clinical supervisors. However, as stakeholders pointed out, individuals are often promoted to supervisory positions without management training or specifically defined roles.

Lifelong learning that builds the competencies of clinical supervisors is essential. Supervisors need training to develop their management skills and to update their competencies as new practices emerge. Competency-based training must acknowledge supervisors' varying skill levels. The Treatment Improvement Protocols (TIPs) developed by SAMHSA have long served as a tool to support the development of competencies and the adoption of specific practices. To further address these diverse training needs, a work group supported by SAMHSA is developing core competency guidelines for clinical supervision. Realizing this tremendous need, several Addiction Technology Transfer Centers (ATTCs) have begun enhancing the skills of clinical supervisors through technology transfer efforts. ATTCs should continue to enhance such efforts, providing ongoing training on clinical supervision based on the core competencies.

In addition to their other functions, clinical supervisors are instrumental in the retention of staff. A recent study of addictions treatment professionals with three or fewer years of experience (NAADAC, 2003) underscores the importance of clinical supervision in promoting job satisfaction and in retaining new frontline workers. This study identified the professional development resources and materials staff found most helpful, and found that staff preferred resources involving interpersonal interaction (e.g., internships, on-the-job training, supervision and mentoring) to more formal written or didactic resources. More than 80 percent of these early-career staff identified clinical supervision as having the greatest value in their professional development (NAADAC, 2003).

Additionally, recovery support supervisors should receive ongoing training. Although the training needs of supervisory staff in recovery support settings are different from those of treatment personnel, they both share a common goal, supporting an individual's recovery. Training should be specifically designed and based on the functions and roles of staff in recovery support positions. The development of such training will require a careful study of recovery support services, the delineation of key categories of services and approaches, and the development of curricula that meet the needs of supervisors guiding the provision of such services. Over time, it would be beneficial to develop core competencies for certain categories of recovery support providers.

SAMHSA/CSAT and the ATTCs, in partnership with recovery support providers, should develop and disseminate core competencies for recovery support supervisors.

2. Develop, Deliver and Sustain Leadership and Management Development Initiatives

Many agency directors are approaching retirement age within the next decade and considerable turnover is occurring at high levels of treatment organizations. New leaders and managers are needed to effectively guide increasingly complex delivery systems. Leadership and management practices impact all aspects of the organization: fiscal, clinical, administrative and human resources. Good management practices positively impact retention by maintaining staff, supporting organizational change and fostering increased productivity. They are also critical to maintaining pace in a challenging treatment environment.

For example, organizations frequently diversify funding to offer comprehensive care to patients/clients. Multiple funding streams generate numerous regulatory requirements that must be implemented and monitored by highly skilled managers. This progressively complicated treatment environment necessitates strong management practices. Therefore, it is recommended that leadership and management development initiatives be delivered and sustained for the addictions treatment field.

Discussion

Many changes have occurred since the current generation of leaders entered the field. As co-morbid medical and mental health disorders are identified with increasing frequency among those served, the provision of treatment has become more complex, requiring the participation of multiple disciplines. Science has taken on a more prominent role as the basis for addictions practices and there is a greater focus on outcomes and accountability. As the addictions treatment field grows, the need for effective leadership has never been greater.

Leadership development initiatives must be established and sustained to build the human capacity necessary to manage the organizational and system demands on the workforce. One example of such an initiative is the series of Leadership Institutes funded by SAMHSA through the Partners for Recovery (PFR) initiative and the Addiction Technology Transfer Centers (ATTCs). Incorporating the immersion training developed by the Graduate School of the U.S. Department of Agriculture, these six-month institutes provide a viable model for broad-scale leadership development.

As in any industry, active staff development and succession planning to prepare a new generation of leaders are critical to organizational survival. Most organizations that provide addictions treatment services do not have a coordinated plan to manage existing and future gaps in leadership. Required leadership skills have become more complex and include strategic planning; fiscal planning; an understanding of Federal, State and local policies; and contracting, communications (e.g., public speaking) and collaboration skills and mentoring.

As in all business enterprises, managers must have skills in financing, contracting, team building, marketing and human resource development to operate an organization effectively. Health care organizations' survival is heavily dependent on proven business practices. Many treatment agencies struggle to meet system demands when their managers lack strong business skills. A body of knowledge has begun to develop around best practices that will assist treatment agencies.

Introducing and fostering the use of leadership and management best practices can result in better-run facilities. Management best practices include:

- Providing staff development/training;
- Allowing for flexible work schedules;
- Rotating staff assignments;
- Providing staff mentors;
- Rewarding staff for performance; and
- Providing supportive supervision and manageable caseloads (Annie E. Casey Foundation, 2003; Hager and Brudney, 2004).

A study (Knudsen et al., 2003) suggests good management practices that can improve staff retention and reduce turnover. These include:

- Increased job autonomy;
- Recognition and reward for strong job performance; and
- Establishing a work environment that supports creativity and innovation.

To address the dilemma posed by a lack of business and leadership skills among staff responsible for managing treatment programs, it is recommended that SAMHSA/CSAT continue to support and expand initiatives, such as the Leadership Institutes funded through the PFR initiative and the ATTCs. In addition, States and providers should establish initiatives to foster the development of business skills among staff and to assist providers in developing effective business processes. *The Network for the Improvement of Addiction Treatment* (NIATx), a partnership between the SAMHSA/CSAT *Strengthening Treatment Access and Retention* (STAR) program, the Robert Wood Johnson Foundation's *Paths to Recovery* program, and a number of independent addictions treatment organizations, provides a good example of an initiative that addresses business processes. SAMHSA/CSAT should continue to support such activities.

C. Recruitment Priorities

Recruitment Issues in Brief

The ability to maintain an adequate addictions treatment workforce is threatened by the difficulty in recruiting staff. The Bureau of Labor Statistics estimates that there will be 3,000 unfilled positions for addictions counselors by the year 2010 (Landis et al., 2002). Concurrently, as noted above, NASADAD projects that the need for treatment staff with graduate degrees will increase by 35% by 2010 (NASADAD, 2003). Another study reports that 5,000 new counselors will be needed each year to replace those leaving the workforce (Lewin-VHI, 1994). In addition, stakeholders offer anecdotal information indicating that staffing shortages exist at every level of the workforce. Demographic changes, particularly the aging of the current workforce, are expected to worsen these shortages over the next decade.

Innovative and comprehensive recruitment strategies are needed, such as a loan forgiveness and repayment program, described previously in Section 2, Part A. These strategies must accommodate the dynamic nature of the treatment field, including increased demand for treatment services, the need to keep pace with scientific advances, staff turnover and required training time for staff. Recruitment efforts must also address the underlying conditions that make people reluctant to enter the addictions treatment workforce: low salaries, minimal benefits, negative public perceptions of the field, high caseloads, patients' increasingly complex health care needs, low professional status and stressful working conditions (Knudsen and Gabriel, 2003).

Treatment agencies compete with other sectors of the economy that often pay higher wages and place fewer demands on workers' time. The need for staff with higher levels of education and training is greater now than it was even a few years ago due to the (1) increasing complexity of the patient/client population entering treatment and (2) scientific advances in treatment. The pool of trained workers is failing to keep up with demand. Compounding these issues is the limited supply of new workers. Between 2000 and 2030, for example, the total population of working-age individuals (18 to 64 years) is projected to grow by only 16 percent (Scanlon, 2001).

Staff recruitment is therefore taking on greater urgency in the addictions treatment field. Unquestionably, the issues exacerbating staff recruitment problems are complex and difficult to resolve. The field is challenged with developing creative strategies that address these recruitment issues and must work in partnership with educational institutions, Federal and State agencies, the public health care system, the media and others to develop and implement effective strategies.

Key strategies should be developed for increasing the diversity of the addictions treatment workforce so that it more closely reflects the patient/client population. As Figure 3. (below) shows, there are discrepancies between the demographics of the addictions treatment staff and the addictions treatment patients/clients. Clinicians tend to be White females over the age of 45, while most patients/clients are younger males with more diverse racial and ethnic backgrounds. The addictions treatment workforce must become more diverse and culturally competent at all levels to better serve the patient/client population (Kaplan, 2003).

	Clinicians	**Patients**
Age	Average age: 45-50	50% between ages 25-44
Race	70-90% Non-Hispanic Whites	60% Non-Hispanic Whites
Gender	50-70% Female	70% Male Admissions

Source: Kaplan, 2003; SAMHSA, 2002.

Figure 3. Demographics of the Workforce.

Recommendations

Stakeholders made the following recommendations:

1. Expand recruitment of health care professionals in addictions medicine;
2. Improve student recruitment with educational institutions, focusing on under-represented groups;
3. Employ marketing strategies to attract workers to the addictions treatment field; and
4. Continue efforts to reduce the stigma associated with working in addictions treatment.

1. Expand Recruitment of Health Care Professionals in Addictions Medicine

The tremendous growth over the past two decades in the availability of medications in substance use disorder treatment, and the increasingly complicated medical conditions that the patient/client population brings to treatment, reaffirm the need for more nurses, physicians and psychiatrists in specialty treatment. Few programs, other than those that offer methadone as an adjunct to treatment, have nurses on staff and just over half employ physicians (McLellan et al., 2003).

Discussion

Some of the boundaries that have traditionally separated specialty addictions and generalist medicine need to become substantially more porous in order to permit the development of strong workforces and truly responsive care systems. Generally, strategies need to be developed to attract larger numbers of physicians to addictions medicine and to encourage larger numbers of nurses and medical social workers to obtain addictions certification. As Figure 4. shows, a relatively small percentage of physicians, nurses and other health professionals obtain addictions credentials or self-identify as an addictions specialist.

Discipline	Workforce Size	Certified Addictions Specialists
Primary care	700,000	2,790 ASAM certified
Psychiatry	30,000	1,067 addictions psychiatrists
Clinical Psychology	69,800	950 APA substance abuse certified
Social Work	300,000	29,400*
Nursing	2,200,000	4,100*
Physician assistant	27,500	185*
Marriage/family therapy	50,000	2,500*

*Self-described addictions specialist.
Source: IOM, 1997.

Figure 4. Number of Practitioners and Certified Addictions Specialists, by Health Care Discipline.

In the short term, recruitment strategies need to begin with professional associations, credentialing bodies and the institutions of higher learning and teaching hospitals where physicians, nurses, social workers, psychologists and other allied professionals are trained. Physicians, psychiatrists, nurses and other medical providers must be recruited within the generalist setting to provide a variety of care, including SBIRT, primary health care and mental health services. There is a critical need for cross-fertilization and cross-training. Specialists and generalists in substance use disorders need to establish care networks and otherwise collaborate to build systems of care that can effectively address the full spectrum of substance use problems, ranging from hazardous use to dependence with co-occurring medical and mental health disorders.

Figure 4. contains data from a 1997 IOM report that compares the number of practitioners by professional discipline to the subset of those same practitioners who have received specialized addictions certification. These data indicate that only a small number of individuals within the total health care workforce are certified as addictions practitioners. The numbers clearly illustrate the need to develop incentives and opportunities that will increase the number of practicing certified addictions treatment professionals. Increased use of medications alone requires additional physicians and nurses to prescribe, administer, monitor and manage patient care.

To support the recruitment and training of medical personnel, a loan forgiveness and repayment program, such as the one proposed in *Infrastructure Development Priorities*, should make loan payment available to medical practitioners who specialize in addictive disorders and agree to work for a specified period of time in publicly funded programs targeting under-served communities. Such a program would encourage specialization of medical practitioners in addictions within both the generalist and specialist settings. The target audience for this special incentive would include physicians, advanced practice nurses, registered nurses and physician assistants who have large student loan obligations, and who desire additional formal training and certification to develop expertise and clinical practice in addictions treatment. It is recommended that marketing strategies and materials target experienced professionals who work in areas such as general internal medicine, family practice, pediatrics, cardiology, geriatrics and other medical specialties.

2. Improve Student Recruitment with Educational Institutions, Focusing on Underrepresented Groups

Student recruitment, at various age levels, is needed to expand the addictions treatment workforce. It is recommended that SAMHSA provide Federal leadership and partner with elementary schools, middle schools, high schools and institutions of higher learning to generate early student interest and to promote opportunities within the field. In particular, recruitment should focus on students with diverse racial and ethnic backgrounds and males to achieve a greater balance between the treatment clinicians and patients/clients. As noted above (see Figure 3.), data show that minorities are under-represented and females are over-represented in the addictions treatment workforce relative to the patient/client population.

Discussion

For marked expansion of the addictions workforce to occur, a much younger cohort must be inspired to choose the addictions treatment field as a career. Educators report that students form opinions as early as fifth grade about careers that they deem desirable (Bell and Ginsburg, 2004). Young people must be exposed to information about the field so that they are aware that it is a viable career option later in life. It is also important to give students early, positive and clear images of the field to counter negative stereotypes and misperceptions they may have developed or encountered. Educational efforts should begin as early as elementary school, continuing through middle school and high school. Recruitment activities should begin in high school and continue through post-graduate education.

Any student recruitment effort must seek to create a more diverse workforce to ensure culturally competent care and to reduce health disparities. *Healthy People 2010* maintains that "increasing the number of minority health professionals is ... a partial solution to improving access to care" (DHHS, 2000). Paraphrasing one of the key conclusions of the Institute of Medicine's report, *In the Nation's Compelling Interest: Ensuring Diversity in the Health Care Workforce* (2004), IOM member Brian Smedley stated: "Part of a comprehensive strategy to reduce health disparities is to increase diversity in the health care professions, which will lead to improved access to care, greater patient satisfaction and reduced cultural and linguistic barriers" (Levin, 2004).

Specifically, it is recommended that SAMHSA partner with educational institutions to collaboratively devise comprehensive recruitment strategies. These strategies must include the development of informational materials about the field for teachers, guidance counselors and librarians. Additionally, support should be made available for mentoring programs, internships, apprenticeships, educational scholarships, loan forgiveness and repayment programs and postgraduate job placement opportunities.

3. Employ Marketing Strategies to Attract Workers to the Addictions Treatment Field

Federal agencies could significantly enhance recruiting efforts by developing model social marketing and health communication strategies aimed at a more diverse group of professionals. Key groups that could be targeted include students, who might be encouraged to adopt addictions treatment as a career path, second-career professionals, individuals in recovery and their family members and other groups that have a natural interest in the field. The recruitment of students and young adults is critical to the development and long-term sustainability of the field.

Discussion

Nursing and other professions have made effective use of the media to recruit workers. For example, an intensive multi-year campaign to attract individuals to nursing was implemented in 2002 (Johnson & Johnson, 2003). One year later, after years of declining enrollment, nursing schools began to experience an increase in the number of applicants and in enrollment.

The addictions treatment field should adopt similar strategies with the anticipation of seeing comparable results. Using basic principles of health communication and social marketing, the field should develop targeted, consumer-centered messages through deliberate placement of advertising designed to reach specific audience segments, including young people and minorities, to create diverse applicant pools. To support this, SAMHSA/CSAT should develop model social marketing and health communications strategies that States and providers can use as models. All media options and recruitment channels (e.g., employee referrals, job fairs, classified advertising, links with educational institutions and online job sites) should be explored. As noted above, it will be critically important to recruit younger individuals who are interested in finding a long-term career path in addictions treatment. Over the long term it is through young persons who elect to make addictions treatment a career that the field will develop most fully as a unique profession.

Second-career professionals, while potentially having a shorter career span, bring maturity, broad life and work experience to the field that is extremely valuable. Those in recovery and their family members, of course, have long brought unique, first-hand experience, passion and perspective to the field. They represent an immense pool of potential workers whose talents would provide an immeasurable benefit to the field. Stakeholders have pointed out that, while such individuals already represent a significant segment of the addictions treatment workforce, the field has barely begun to tap this rich resource.

4. Continue Efforts to Reduce the Stigma Associated with Working in Addictions Treatment

Stigma devalues addictions treatment as a meaningful career and reduces the size of the prospective labor pool, making staff recruitment difficult. Drawing from best practices in other fields such as nursing, SAMHSA/CSAT leadership should be provided to develop strategies, including a public education campaign, to promote addictions treatment as a worthwhile career choice.

Discussion

Workforce recruitment efforts must overcome the stigmatization of the addictions treatment field. Other health professions, like nursing, have implemented successful initiatives to address stigmatization and its negative impacts, with support from Federal and State agencies. The success of stigma reduction efforts has instilled the nursing profession with a more positive self-image and shown nurses to be a valuable and necessary national resource.

The nursing profession has approached the issue of stigma and its workforce crisis in a variety of ways (Nevidjon and Erickson, 2001). It has:

- Worked to define and distinguish the profession through research, education and clinical service;
- Engaged professional nursing associations as advocates to gain support and recognition;
- Obtained support from professional colleagues (e.g., doctors); and
- Challenged the media to present positive and true images of the nursing profession (Donley et al., 2002).

Although negative images and stigma associated with nursing have not disappeared entirely and a nursing shortage still exists, progress has been made. A study by Bacon, MacKenzie and McKendrick (2000), for example, found that nurses are now viewed as well-educated, independent thinkers who play a key role within a high-tech medical world. This improved image has enabled the field to recruit more young people and career-minded professionals.

These strategies provide examples of what could be accomplished in the addictions treatment field. However, additional approaches, such as the development of a national campaign to educate the public about the scientific basis and effectiveness of addictions treatment, are also necessary. This campaign should:

- Demonstrate the effectiveness of treatment services;
- Bring distinction to the field; and
- Place a human face on recovery.

The written and electronic media, public education system and the health professions should be targets of the campaign. In particular, the campaign should present the addictions treatment field and addictions studies as exciting, viable and respectable career choices and seek to build the public's confidence in the importance and effectiveness of treatment services. It is recommended that SAMHSA/CSAT partner with States, academic institutions, provider trade associations and other stakeholders to explore the feasibility of developing public information campaigns to market careers in addictions treatment.

D. Addictions Education and Accreditation Priorities

Education and Accreditation Issues in Brief

Academic training is fundamental to developing a quality workforce and to providing quality care. Although progress has been made in raising academic standards in addictions studies programs to the level of programs in other health care disciplines, several serious gaps remain.

A significant problem is the lack of education and training on substance use disorders for primary health care and other health and human services professionals. The National Center on Addictions and Substance Abuse (CASA) at Columbia University reported that 94 percent of primary care physicians and 40 percent of pediatricians, when presented with a person with a substance use disorder, failed to diagnose the problem properly (CASA, 2000). If similar studies were available for other health professionals (e.g., nurses, psychologists, pharmacists, social workers, dentists), the results would likely be similar. The primary reason for health professionals' failure to diagnose substance use disorders is a lack of knowledge about the disease. Curricula in most health education programs and professional schools either inadequately address substance use disorders or exclude discussion of them all together.

New demands are being placed on the higher education system as the need for academic training grows within the addictions treatment field. Historically, training for addictions treatment tended to resemble an apprentice model. This model emphasizes experience over formal education. An apprentice model can best be described as training in which the majority of knowledge, skills and ability to practice are imparted through supervision. With the need to treat and manage complex patients/clients and implement evidenced-based practices in the workplace, the call for more formal education to complement supervision is changing the workforce culture. Increasingly, States are finding the need to require formal education through credentialing and licensure standards (SAMHSA, 2005).

Colleges and universities rely on a variety of standards to develop curricula, rather than one set of national competencies. Although efforts have been made to establish national academic accreditation standards for addictions studies, they have not been adopted. Program accreditation would provide recognition and demonstrate an ongoing commitment to quality education.

Presently, 442 colleges and universities across the country offer addictions studies programs. Eighteen percent are at the graduate level, 13 percent are at the undergraduate level and 69 percent are at the associate level (Taleff, 2003). Anecdotally, information from stakeholders suggests that tremendous variation exists among these academic programs with regard to level of course difficulty, use of evidence-based materials, quality of faculty and ability to prepare students for clinical practice. Additionally, the relevance of coursework and its relationship to research depends greatly on faculty members' abilities to stay current on recently completed and ongoing research.

The changing demographics of the Nation demand a multi-cultural and multi-lingual workforce. Although enrollment remains at record high levels for traditional college-age students, those under 25 years old (Jamieson et al., 2001), data are not available about the number of racial and ethnic minorities enrolled in addictions studies programs, or the progress that has been made to increase minority enrollment.

Recommendations

To improve the academic caliber of education programs for the addictions treatment field, stakeholders made the following recommendations:

1. Include training on addictions as part of education programs for primary health care and for other health and human service professions (e.g., physicians, nurses, psychologists and social workers);
2. Call for the use of national addictions core competencies as the basis of curricula;
3. Support the development and adoption of national accreditation standards for addictions education programs;
4. Encourage national and State boards for the health professions to have at least 10 percent of licensing examination questions pertain to addictions;

5. Support academic programs in Historically Black Colleges and Universities (HBCUs), Hispanic Serving Institutions, Tribal Colleges and Universities and other minority-serving institutions; and
6. Develop college and university courses in addictions-related health services research and its application; and systematically disseminate research findings to academic institutions.

1. Include Training on Addictions As Part of Education Programs for Primary Health Care and for Other Health and Human Service Professions (E.G., Physicians, Nurses, Psychologists and Social Workers)

Primary care physicians and other health professionals frequently are the first point of contact in the health care system, yet they often do not recognize substance use disorders. Education related to substance use disorders must be incorporated in all education programs for medical and health professions in order to raise the skill level of health professionals and to expose individuals to the opportunity to specialize in addictions treatment.

Discussion

Physicians and other health and human service professionals do not receive adequate education on substance use disorders. The absence of education on this issue has many implications for patients/clients. Physicians are failing to detect and diagnose problems, despite evidence supporting the efficacy of early intervention. They are failing to provide brief interventions and to refer patients/clients to specialty programs for care when necessary. These oversights have long-lasting consequences. Action needs to be taken in the early stages of substance use disorders when the potential for treatment success is high and the medical and social costs are low (CASA, 2000; Haack and Alemi, 2002; Saitz et al., 1997).

Failure to diagnose and refer patients with substance use disorders occurs, in large part, because of the lack of academic or other training related to substance use disorders. A national survey of residency program directors in seven medical specialties revealed that only 56 percent of the residency programs surveyed had a required curriculum in preventing and treating alcohol and substance use disorders. The most common barriers to providing training were a lack of time (58%), a lack of faculty expertise (37%) and a lack of institutional support (32%). According to the authors, education programs can be improved by integrating training on addictions into existing residency structures, increasing faculty knowledge and including more questions related to treatment on board examinations (Isaacson et al., 2000).

The U.S. DHHS should support expansion of SAMHSA/HRSA joint education initiatives. An example of such an initiative is Project MAINSTREAM (Multi-Agency Initiative on Substance Abuse Training and Education for America), which was part of the HRSA-Association for Medical Education and Research in Substance Abuse (AMERSA)-SAMHSA/CSAT Interdisciplinary Project to Improve Health Professional Education on Substance Abuse. This and similar programs were designed to enhance substance use disorders training and education among health professionals.

Such programs would benefit social workers. Many clinical social workers are eligible to practice in the addictions treatment field as a result of their social work license, but may lack the specialty education and training that would permit them to provide the most effective care. The curricula of undergraduate schools of social work, for example, vary in the extent to which the treatment of substance use disorders is covered. Some graduate schools of social work offer a concentration in substance use disorders; others offer only elective courses.

A 2000 survey of the members of the National Association of Social Workers by the Practice Research Network (PRN) Project found that only 38 percent of members had completed formal coursework in substance use disorder treatment during their academic programs, and 87 percent indicated that they held no certification in the treatment of substance use disorders (NASW PRN, 2001). Academic institutions, in partnership with professional organizations, should develop enhanced multi- and cross-disciplinary education and training programs to provide core curricula for social workers and health professionals on substance use disorders.

2. Call for the Use of National Addictions Core Competencies As the Basis of Curricula

Educational curricula must be based on solid research and on a unified national set of core competencies to prepare a workforce that is both knowledgeable and skilled. A unified standard must be created within the higher education system based on core competencies identified by experts in the substance use disorder field. SAMHSA Technical Assistance Protocol (TAP) 21, *Addiction Counseling Competencies: The Knowledge, Skills and Attitudes of Professional Practice,* includes some of the best thinking in the country on this topic and is recommended as the basis for curricula development.

Discussion

Educational institutions use a number of standards when developing curricula. These standards include the International Certification and Reciprocity Consortium (IC&RC) twelve core functions; the International Coalition for Addictions Studies Education (INCASE) standards; the Association for Addiction Professionals (NAADAC) Certification Standards; and SAMHSA TAP 21.

The lack of consistency in academic curricula works to the detriment of the field. Many treatment professionals and organizations agree that TAP 21 should be the basis for curriculum development. TAP 21 is designed to impart the knowledge, skills and attitudes for achieving and practicing addictions counseling competencies.

Key entities that have endorsed the publication include the National Association of State Alcohol and Drug Abuse Directors (NASADAD), NAADAC, IC&RC and several States. TAP 21 focuses on two broad themes:

- The **knowledge and attitudes** underlying competent practice for both addictions treatment counselors and practitioners in other disciplines: understanding addictions, treatment knowledge, application of knowledge to practice and professional readiness; and
- **Clinical skills and competencies**, including: evaluation, treatment planning, referral, service coordination, counseling, patient/client interactions, family and community education, documentation and professional and ethical responsibilities.

Focusing curricula on competencies is essential to ensure that students leaving the academic community possess not only the knowledge they need, but also the skills and behaviors necessary to prepare them for clinical practice. Developing curricula based on core competencies ensures that students leaving the academic setting have a common set of knowledge and skills to provide appropriate and effective treatment services. Institutions of higher education should use national core competencies as the basis of curricula.

3. Support the Development and Adoption of National Accreditation Standards for Addictions Education Programs

There is no uniform national programmatic structure nor are there associated standards for addictions studies despite the existence of 442 addictions studies programs across the United States. Little is known about the quality of these programs and how they prepare future practitioners. Academic accreditation standards for addictions studies programs need to be developed, adopted and supported.

Discussion

> "Accreditation standards would give programs a greater degree of professionalism, would provide consistency and would standardize substance abuse education curricula" (PFR Meeting of College and University Faculty, 2004).

Academic accreditation standards should be adopted to improve the quality and standing of addictions education programs. Educators in addictions studies expressed the feeling that their programs were given "second class" status by their institutions. Accreditation has advantages for educators as well as students. Educators gain access to a network of other accredited programs for sharing best practices and professional knowledge. Faculty members participate in peer review processes. Students benefit from an enriched environment for learning and greater ease in transitioning credits from one accredited school to another.

INCASE is developing accreditation standards for college and university addictions education programs. Several related issues will need to be considered as the process moves forward. First, addictions studies educators state that there is a shortage of qualified faculty, although data are needed to further substantiate this. A second issue is that many faculty members do not have terminal degrees and would therefore need access to doctoral programs. A third issue is that most programs in addictions counseling are at the associate degree level and no accreditation bodies currently recognize associate degree level programs. When implemented, accreditation standards will assist schools in developing new addictions studies programs and will enhance the reputation of existing programs that compete for students and institutional support.

It is recommended that SAMHSA/CSAT partner with institutions of higher education to foster adoption of national accreditation standards for addictions studies.

4. Encourage National and State Boards for the Health Professions to Have at Least 10 Percent of Licensing Examination Questions Pertain to Addictions

Representatives of licensure, certification and accreditation bodies in the health professions should enhance the content of their testing requirements to reflect key knowledge and concepts related to the treatment of addictions, by ensuring that at least 10 percent of questions pertain to substance use disorders.

Discussion

The core curriculum in the health professions is strongly influenced by licensing examinations and certification requirements. If items on the treatment of addictions were included in the licensing and certification examinations, the topic of addictions would receive more emphasis in the core curriculum of each discipline in the field (Haack and Adger, 2002).

Licensing and certification examinations could include questions relevant to methods of screening; brief intervention; motivational interviewing; pharmacotherapy and psychosocial interventions for relapse prevention; treating and referring for co-morbid medical and psychiatric conditions; recognizing and referring professional colleagues impaired by substance use; legal and ethical issues related to serving individuals with hazardous or dependent substance use patterns and a variety of other topics deemed appropriate by governing licensure and accreditation boards (Haack and Adger, 2002). For certain specialists whose licensing requirements include oral examinations, State licensing boards should also include competency content in the area of addictions. The addition of these questions to licensing and certification examinations will aid in ensuring that candidates are competent to recognize and treat addictions.

Federal agencies, in partnership with private and public organizations, should take the lead in bringing this issue to the attention of key organizations with which they interact. Groups that should collaborate in this effort include national, State and discipline-specific organizations related to licensure, certification and accreditation of medical and nursing professionals and the licensing and accrediting bodies of other disciplines in the health professions (Haack and Adger, 2002). Implementation of this recommendation will help create a standard of care for health care professionals serving individuals with addictions, as well as create criteria for evaluating programs that prepare these professionals to take licensure and certification examinations.

State addictions treatment authorities should work with licensing bodies to ensure that 10% of licensing questions pertain to addictions. To accomplish this, they will also need to work with institutions of higher education, to encourage development of curricula that prepare future professionals to address addictions.

5. Support Academic Programs in Historically Black Colleges and Universities (Hbcus), Hispanic Serving Institutions, Tribal Colleges and Universities and Other Minority-Serving Institutions

Nationally, racial and ethnic minorities are projected to grow from 28 percent of the population in 2000 to nearly 40 percent by 2030 (Dochterman and Grace, 2001). The multicultural composition of the population requires that greater attention be given to diversifying the workforce. A significant disparity already exists between clinicians and patients/clients in the addictions treatment field. Providing support for educational programs targeting racial and ethnic minorities will ultimately result in more graduates who will become part of the treatment workforce.

Academic programs that support racial and ethnic minority students offer great promise for addressing unmet health care needs. Initiatives supporting curriculum development, internships, apprenticeships, loan forgiveness and scholarships at academic institutions that serve minority populations would provide a mechanism to increase the diversity of the workforce and provide care in underserved areas (DHHS/HRSA, 2004).

Discussion

HBCUs and other minority-serving institutions should develop additional coursework and curricula in addictions studies. Greater variation in coursework makes programs more attractive to students, encouraging them to consider addictions studies. Internships and apprenticeship programs are also critical components in the development of clinicians. States and provider organizations should support paid internships and apprenticeships as a means of providing students with practical experience that can lead to future employment.

One of the most effective incentives for recruiting young people into the field is a loan forgiveness and repayment program. The loan forgiveness and repayment program proposed in *Infrastructure Development Priorities* would be instrumental in supporting recruitment from HBCUs and other minority-serving institutions. Such a program could be an effective mechanism for recruiting young, culturally diverse staff. Loan forgiveness alleviates the significant financial burden associated with obtaining professional staff credentials. Typically, a service requirement is met in lieu of payment. This benefits both the student and the workforce.

The steady growth in the number of racial and ethnic minorities requires an investment of resources to provide greater access and quality of care to these populations. A report by HRSA indicates that minority physicians are more likely to practice in urban areas that experience a shortage of services, thereby increasing access to services for minority and medically underserved communities (HRSA, 2003). Thus, support for addictions studies programs at HBCUs, Hispanic Serving Institutions, Tribal Colleges and Universities and other minority-serving institutions is needed to ensure workforce diversity and respond to the treatment needs of these diverse populations.

6. Develop College and University Courses in Addictions-Related Health Services Research and Its Application; and Systematically Disseminate Research Findings to Academic Institutions

One of the greatest challenges for the addictions treatment field is the dissemination and institutionalization of evidence-based practices. NIDA and NIAAA have conducted considerable research in substance use disorders. However, systematic mechanisms do not currently exist to disseminate research findings to academic institutions. No mechanisms exist to ensure that the most current research informs educational practices.

Implementing evidence-based practices requires a workforce trained to understand how to find and use new knowledge. As clearly noted in the IOM's report on *Crossing the Quality Chasm* (2001), clinical education needs to include courses on evidence-based practices and on learning how to access, understand and use research. Therefore, addictions studies programs at colleges and universities must include courses that teach students about research and how to apply it in practice.

Discussion

The addictions treatment field's focus on evidence-based practice and patient/client outcomes requires a workforce equipped to be lifelong learners and accustomed to incorporating research findings in practice. Pre-service education should include required courses on understanding and applying these principles. As accreditation standards for addictions studies programs are developed, basic courses on research design, terminology, statistics and program fidelity should be a part of the required curriculum.

Over the past three decades, NIDA and NIAAA have supported rigorous research that has informed our understanding of substance use disorders and treatment. Unfortunately, many research findings have not reached the educator or practitioner and therefore have not influenced addictions education or treatment practice. It is essential that faculty remain current on research findings, so that students receive information on the latest treatment technology and science. Therefore, it is recommended that NIDA and NIAAA disseminate research findings to colleges and universities, particularly to those offering addictions studies programs.

E. Retention Priorities

Retention Issues in Brief

Nearly 70 percent (67.8%) of addictions treatment staff have worked with their current employer for five years or less (Harwood, 2002). Data from the University of Georgia National Treatment Center Study indicate an average annual turnover rate of 18.5 percent among addictions treatment counselors. This rate far exceeds the national average of 11 percent across all occupations and is significantly higher than the average annual turnover rates for teachers (13%) and nurses (12%), occupations traditionally known to have high staff turnover (Knudsen et al., 2003).

Maintaining a stable workforce is the goal of every profession. Such stability helps ensure continuity, quality of care and a positive work environment. Turnover is minimized when individuals experience a high level of job satisfaction and are committed to staying in the profession. Low salaries, lack of career paths, insufficient mentorship programs, inadequate staff supervision, personnel shortages and large caseloads contribute to staff turnover and job discontent in the addictions treatment field.

The negative impact and costs of employee turnover are well documented. In testimony before the Senate Committee on Health, Education, Labor and Pensions, William J. Scanlon, Director of Health Care Issues at the Government Accountability Office (GAO), discussed the problem of turnover in the nursing profession (Scanlon, 2001). Many of the issues Scanlon raised also pertain to the addictions treatment workforce. Specifically, Scanlon identified the following costs related to staff turnover:

- Time and expense of recruitment, selection and training of new staff;
- Inefficiencies related to entry of new staff;
- Decreased group morale and productivity; and
- Disrupted continuity of patient care.

Retention efforts must be creative, innovative and address underlying reasons that cause individuals to quit their jobs or leave the field. Career path development, training on clinical supervision, leadership and management development and marketing of the field have been discussed earlier in this report and are potential retention strategies.

Recommendations

Stakeholders made the following additional recommendations to develop a multi-faceted retention strategy to improve workforce retention:

1. Identify and disseminate best practices in staff retention; and
2. Address substance misuse and relapse within the workforce.

1. Identify and Disseminate Best Practices in Staff Retention

National leadership should be provided regarding the identification and dissemination of best practices related to salary structure and benefits, financial incentives, continuing education, alternative work schedules, mentoring, employee wellness practices and professional advancement. Dissemination of practices to State Directors, providers, ATTCs and professional and trade associations within the addictions treatment field should be a major priority.

Discussion

> "Turnover takes away the most valuable resource that the field has: the knowledge and experience needed to help clients achieve recovery" (The Lewin Group, 2004).

When retention rates are low and turnover is high, facility operations and patient/client care are compromised. Low salaries contribute to high turnover. Salaries of individuals working in the addictions treatment field are not competitive compared to those of other health professionals in equivalent job categories. Figure 5. provides information on the median annual earnings for addictions treatment counselors and other health and social service providers by occupation in 2000.

The U.S. Department of Labor reports that in 2000 the median income for addictions treatment and behavioral disorder counselors was $28,510. As of 2000, the mean annual salary for all addictions treatment counselors in the United States was $30,100. The region with the most counselors (mid-Atlantic) had the highest mean annual salary at $34,433 per year. While the mean annual salaries for addictions treatment counselors are comparatively low across the regions, the cost of living varies greatly by region. In many regions, salaries place many workers at bare subsistence. Additionally, a survey of addictions treatment counselors found that 30 percent had no medical coverage, 40 percent had no dental coverage and 55 percent were not covered for substance use or mental health services (Galfano, 2004).

Occupation	Median Annual Earnings ($)	Occupation	Median Annual Earnings ($)
Rehabilitation counselors	24,450	Medical and public health social workers	34,790
Mental health counselors	27,570	Educational, vocational and school counselors	42,110
Substance abuse and behavioral disorder counselors	28,510	Registered nurses	44,480
Licensed practical and vocational nurses	29,440	Psychologists (clinical, counseling and school)	48,320
Mental health and substance abuse social workers	30,170	Physician assistants	61,910
Child, family and school social workers	31,470	Family and general practitioners	130,000*
Marriage and family therapists	34,660	Psychiatrists	130,000*

Source: U.S. Department of Labor, 2003 and, when indicated by an asterisk (*), the American Medical Association.

Figure 5. Median Annual Earnings of Community and Social Service Counselors and Selected Behavioral Health Professionals in 2000.

A 2003 study of individuals in the addictions treatment workforce found that the most prevalent recommendation for retaining staff was increasing salaries (Knudsen and Gabriel, 2003). In addition, other financial incentives such as bonuses and performance awards aid in retention. Employees who perceive that their organizations provide them with more rewarding and supportive environments are more likely to be committed to the organization. Therefore, as the field develops a multi-faceted strategy for workforce retention, it is recommended that SAMHSA identify and disseminate to the States best practices related to workforce compensation and financial incentives and support strategic planning needed to implement a national workforce retention effort.

Private sector research also suggests that management practices and organizational commitments that (1) increase job autonomy and accountability for workers, (2) support creativity and new ideas and (3) provide non-tangible rewards linked to performance may improve addictions workforce retention

(Knudsen et al., 2003). According to research in the public sector, good management practices that offer employee training, reduce paperwork, increase individual recognition, promote career growth and improve the physical work environment enhance retention (Knudsen and Gabriel, 2003). Creating a work environment that values and empowers all employees is vital.

Anecdotal evidence indicates that recruitment and retention problems associated with faculty for addictions studies programs are just as severe as those seen in the rest of the workforce. (At the present time, adequate data are not available on the academic workforce.) The challenges involved in recruiting faculty for addictions studies programs in turn makes it increasingly difficult to recruit, develop and certify degreed treatment professionals. As part of a multifaceted strategy to recruit addictions program faculty, experienced treatment professionals who are at risk of leaving the field should be offered the opportunity to participate in specially designed accelerated degree programs (i.e., Master's or Doctorate) or other training enabling them to become addictions treatment faculty at institutions of higher learning. With support from SAMHSA, Federal and State government agencies and colleges and universities should develop a pilot project to recruit addictions studies faculty. A successful pilot would establish a "promising practice" for workforce retention.

2. Address Substance Misuse and Relapse within the Workforce

To date, little attention has been given to the issue of substance misuse and relapse in the workforce. Leadership is required in this area. The Addiction Technology Transfer Centers (ATTCs), in partnership with clinicians, treatment providers, States and other stakeholders, can lead the development of training that recognizes and addresses substance misuse and relapse within the workforce. Training areas should include, but not be limited to, strengthening Employee Assistance Programs (EAPs), wellness programs and health insurance and disability policies. Such training would target supervisors, human resource managers, the general provider workforce and State/Territory agency staff.

Discussion

While all professions employ individuals in recovery, the addictions treatment field is unusual in the proportion of its workforce that is in recovery. It is unique in that many of the recovering individuals among its ranks work in the same health care system through which they received treatment. Anecdotally, the numbers of recovering individuals entering the treatment workforce may be decreasing, but the percentages are still significant by treatment agency estimates. The potential for relapse is always present, even among addictions specialists. While relapse is most likely during the first four to five years of abstinence, it can occur at any stage of the recovery process. Individuals in recovery are an invaluable resource to the field because they bring insight from personal experience, passion and commitment to their work. In addition, substance misuse among clinicians and other treatment staff who may not have a diagnosable substance use disorder must also be addressed. EAPs are one mechanism for addressing this.

Small agencies often do not have adequate resources to offer EAP services to their employees and often are only able to provide very limited health and disability benefits. Wellness programs may offer an effective strategy for such agencies. They "have the potential to decrease absenteeism, reduce medical claims costs, and improve employee productivity, recruitment, and retention" and can be implemented inexpensively by smaller organizations (Sullivan, 2000). While not necessarily representing a direct response to relapse or substance use, a wellness program could serve as both a preventive measure and a support to interventions more specifically targeted to substance misuse and relapse in the workforce.

Clinicians face the reality of relapse every day in managing patients/clients, but many treatment agencies are not well prepared to address relapse within their own staff. Moreover, detection of a substance use disorder and relapse is often delayed by the ability of individuals to protect their job performance at the expense of every other aspect of their lives (Brown et al., 2002). Many organizations lack policies and resources that assist supervisors in taking appropriate action when impairment is detected. Organizations shy away from human resource policies covering these situations due to liability, financial concerns and fears of disclosure. A relapse prevention strategy for managers and staff is needed for treatment organizations, as well as general training for referring employees for assistance related to a substance use problem. The ATTCs, in partnership with States, provider organizations and other stakeholders, should develop and conduct training for human resource departments, supervisory and management staff and clinicians related to substance misuse and relapse prevention strategies.

Additionally, it is recommended that SAMHSA fund the piloting of an impaired professionals' program for addictions clinicians to determine whether, when and under what circumstances a clinician who has relapsed can re-enter direct clinical practice. While it may not be possible for a clinician to resume the provision of direct services immediately after a relapse, it may be possible to establish systems and supports that will enable the clinician to return to the provision of services within a reasonable period of time. A pilot could yield preliminary standards for the field. Such a program would interface with the EAP and the treatment agency human resources department. Lastly, provider organizations should train staff on how and when to refer colleagues for assistance when they suspect misuse of substances.

Data from the medical profession indicate that such programs can be quite effective. One study compared 73 physicians who received ongoing monitoring after treatment in an inpatient setting to 185 middle managers who were treated but not monitored. It found that 83 percent of the physicians had favorable outcomes compared to 62 percent of the managers. The researchers hypothesized that the close monitoring received by the physicians accounted for the better outcomes. In addition, a study of 63 impaired or addicted physicians put on probation by the Oregon Health Board found that, of the subset that was monitored, 96 percent remained abstinent whereas only 64 percent of the subset that was not monitored had remained abstinent (Brown et al., 2002).

Any existing programs serving professionals working in the addictions treatment field should be identified, and the national, State and local certification boards or professional societies for addictions treatment professionals should be encouraged to explore development of peer education and support programs for impaired professionals in the addictions treatment field. Relapse within the addictions treatment workforce presents the field with significant challenges. However, the development of relapse prevention strategies, relevant policies and procedures and impaired professional and peer education programs would provide tools to respond systematically and effectively to this challenge.

F. Study Priorities

Study Issues in Brief

Data on the addictions treatment workforce have been limited. A number of ATTCs have conducted surveys of the treatment workforce (Knudsen and Gabriel, 2003; Gallon et al., 2003). The surveys, which differ in content and methodology, focus on issues such as academic training and professional experience, recruitment and retention, compensation, treatment models, training interests and employee satisfaction. While informative, such studies do not yield data to guide the development of the addictions treatment workforce.

Addictions treatment would benefit from research data that show the relationship between the education, training and demographic characteristics of treatment professionals and patient/client outcomes. These research findings would enable the field to make informed decisions about professional development and improved practices.

Recommendations

The list of study topics related to workforce development is potentially long. Many questions specific to workforce competencies, workforce performance and recruitment and retention practice have yet to be answered. However, three topics have been identified by the stakeholders as priorities:

1. Conduct studies that examine the relationships among level of education, type of education, training and treatment outcomes;
2. Conduct studies that examine the relationships among clinician and patient/client cultural, demographic and other characteristics and treatment outcomes; and
3. Conduct studies of clinician characteristics, training and skills that enhance therapeutic alliance.

1. Conduct Studies That Examine the Relationships Among Level of Education, Type of Education, Training and Treatment Outcomes

It is recommended that NIDA and NIAAA fund studies to determine the relationship between a practitioner's level and type of training and specific treatment outcomes. Minimal research currently exists on the impact of education and training on treatment outcomes. Health services research on this topic could provide valuable information to the field by focusing on the following questions:

- Do some types of training produce better treatment outcomes than others?
- What is the relationship between a clinician's education and treatment outcomes?
- Is experiential or academic training of greater value to treatment outcomes?

Discussion

Health services research has provided information on the basic competencies needed to perform certain treatment practices and the types of education and training necessary to support skill development. However, limited research has been conducted on how education and training are linked to treatment outcomes. Such research could help to guide the design of academic and continuing education, faculty development, supervision and technology transfer strategies. Research on the relationship of training and education to treatment outcomes would also provide the field with necessary information for recruitment.

2. Conduct Studies That Examine the Relationships among Clinician and Patient/Client Cultural, Demographic and Other Characteristics and Treatment Outcomes

The disparity in age, gender, race and ethnicity between clinicians and patients/clients has led to increased concerns about the impact of these differences on treatment outcomes. However, little substantive research is available on the effects of an addictions treatment professional's demographic, cultural background and other characteristics on patient/client treatment outcomes.

Health services research is needed to address questions such as:

- Are cultural, demographic and other characteristics of clinicians relevant to improving treatment outcomes? If so, which ones?
- Do learned cultural competency skills improve treatment outcomes?
- Are treatment professionals in recovery more effective?
- Does gender matching affect treatment outcomes? If so, how?

Discussion

Available data show that clinicians are predominantly White women in their mid-forties to early fifties while patients/clients are somewhat younger males from racially and ethnically diverse backgrounds (SAMHSA, 2002; Kaplan, 2003). Although much has been said about the disparities between the demographic characteristics of clinicians and patients/clients, little research has been conducted to date on the impact of these differences on treatment outcomes. Survey data collected by the ATTCs provide general information about workforce demographics and challenges, but shed little light on whether professionals with different educational backgrounds and demographic characteristics contribute differentially to treatment outcomes.

Research on these topics would help human resource personnel to focus recruitment and retention efforts appropriately. This research would also guide student and faculty recruitment, as well as culturally competent and gender-specific curriculum development at educational and training institutions. It is recommended that NIDA and NIAAA fund research examining the relationship between clinician and client cultural, demographic and other characteristics and outcomes.

3. Conduct Studies of Clinician Characteristics, Training and Skills That Enhance Therapeutic Alliance

In the past two decades, a number of studies investigating the role of therapeutic alliance in drug treatment have been published (Meier et al., 2005). This body of literature supports the fact that the relationship skills of the clinician are important in improving patient/client outcomes. An example of another factor that may impact therapeutic alliance is the recovery status of the clinician. Little research has been performed on the relationship between clinician recovery status, therapeutic alliance and outcomes. Therefore, the extent to which the recovery status of clinicians is associated with an effective therapeutic alliance is not well known. As the field strives to improve patient/client outcomes and enhance the skills of its workforce, answers to several research questions would provide valuable information:

- What skills are needed to build a therapeutic alliance?
- Can training improve a practitioner's ability to build a therapeutic alliance?
- What training methods are most effective?
- Is the recovery status of the clinician correlated with the quality of therapeutic alliance?
- Do the philosophy and nature of interventions employed by recovering and non- recovering clinicians vary?

Discussion

A therapeutic alliance refers to the relationship that develops between a patient/client and a clinician. The relationship is often characterized by the emotional bond and trust that occurs between the clinician and patient/client. Among the common elements of psychotherapy, the collaborative relationship between the patient/client and therapist is one of the most important. This alliance is just as important for drug therapy as for psychotherapy (Roy-Byrne, 1996).

For addictions treatment, early therapeutic alliance appears to be a consistent predictor of engagement and retention in care (Meier et al., 2005). Yet, little is known about the characteristics of the clinician that enhance therapeutic alliance and therefore improve patient/client outcomes.

Stoffelmayr and colleagues found that, while a clinician's level of education influenced neither treatment goals nor techniques, recovery status of clinicians was correlated with the range of treatment techniques and treatment goals employed. Clinicians who were in recovery tended to adopt more varied treatment techniques and a broader range of treatment goals (Stoffelmayr, 1999). There is some evidence, therefore, that the recovery status of counselors affects how they approach the provision of treatment services.

Further research is required to better understand the relationship between recovery status of the clinician and therapeutic alliance. A better understanding of these relationships will allow recruitment and training efforts to better target individuals who are likely to be effective clinicians. Research will provide information on what clinical skills and clinician attributes support a quality relationship with the patient/client. It is recommended that NIDA and NIAAA fund research examining the characteristics of clinicians that enhance therapeutic alliance.

References

Addiction Technolgy Transfer Center Network (ATTC), *The Change Book: A Blueprint for Technology Transfer (Second Edition),* (Kansas City, MO: ATTC, 2004).

Adler, K.G., "Why It's Time to Purchase an Electronic Health Record System: The Old Reasons for Holding Off May Have Lost Their Validity," *American Academy of Family Physicians News & Publications*, 2004, *Online*, < http://www.aafp.org/fpm/20041100/43whyi.html>, Nov. 2004.

Annie E. Casey Foundation, *The Unsolved Challenge of System Reform: The Condition of the Frontline Human Services Workforce,* (Baltimore, MD: Annie E. Casey Foundation, 2003).

Bacon, K., K.E. MacKenzie and J.H. McKendrick, "Tomorrow's Nurses?" *Nursing Standard* 14(32), 2000, p. 31.

Bell, E. and S. Ginsburg, "An Evaluation of The University of Connecticut Health Center Health Professions Partnership Initiative," (Bethesda, MD: Abt Associates Inc., 2004).

Brown, M.E., A.M. Trinkoff, A.G. Christen and E.J. Dole, "Impairment Issues for Health Care Professionals: Review and Recommendations," *Substance Abuse: Journal of the Association for Medical Education and Research in Substance Abuse* 23(3), Supplement, 2002, pp. 155-165.

Center on Addictions and Substance Abuse (CASA), *Missed Opportunity: National Survey of Primary Care Physicians and Patients on Substance Abuse*, (New York: CASA, Columbia University, 2000).

Culbreth, J.R., "Clinical Supervision of Substance Abuse Counselors: Current and Preferred Practices," *Journal of Addictions and Offender Counseling* 20(1), 1999, pp. 15-25.

Department of Health and Human Services (DHHS), "Access to Quality Health Care Services," *Healthy People 2010: Understanding and Improving Health*, 2nd ed., (Washington, DC: U.S. Government Printing Office, 2000), *Online*, < http://www.healthypeople.gov/Document/HTML /Volume1/01Access.htm>, March 2005, p. 20.

Department of Health and Human Services/Health Resources and Services Administration (DHHS/HRSA), "Optimizing the Impact of the National Health Service Corps," (Rockville, MD: DHHS, 2004).

Dochterman, J.M. and H.K. Grace, "Overview: Diversity in Nursing," *Nursing*, 2001, pp. 480-482.

Donley, R., M.J. Flaherty, E. Sarsfield, L. Taylor, H. Maloni and E. Flanagan, "What Does the Nurse Reinvestment Act Mean to You?" *Online Journal of Issues in Nursing*, 2002, *Online*, <http://www.nursingworld.org/ojin /topic14/tpc14_5.htm>, January 2005.

Fox, C., "Hearing on Strengthening the Safety Net: Increasing Access to Essential Health Care Services" (HRSA Testimony Before the Senate Committee on Health, Education, Labor and Pensions, Subcommittee on Public Health and Safety, Washington, DC, March 22, 2001).

Galfano, S., "2004 Addictions Treatment Professional Career and Salary Survey," *Counselor: The Magazine for Addictions Professionals*, Vol. 5, 2004, pp. 24-29.

Gallon, S., R. Gabriel and J. Knudsen, "The Toughest Job You'll Ever Love: A Pacific Northwest Treatment Workforce Survey," *Journal of Substance Abuse Treatment* 24(3), 2003, pp. 183-196.

Haack, M.R. and H. Adger, "Strategic Plan for Interdisciplinary Faculty Development: Arming the Nation's Workforce for a New Approach to Substance Use Disorders," *Journal of the Association for Medical Education and Research in Substance Abuse* 23(3), Supplement, (Providence, RI: AMERSA, 2002), pp. 1-21.

Haack, M.R. and F. Alemi, "Strategic Plan for Interdisciplinary Faculty Development: Arming the Nation's Health Professional Workforce for a New Approach to Substance Use Disorders," *Journal of the Association for Medical Education and Research in Substance Abuse* 23(3), Supplement, (Providence, RI: AMERSA, 2002), pp. 95-104.

Hager, M.A. and J.L. Brudney, *Volunteer Management Practices and Retention of Volunteers*, (Washington, DC: The Urban Institute, 2004).

Harwood, H.J., "Survey on Behavioral Health Workplace," *Frontlines: Linking Alcohol Services Research and Practice*, (Bethesda, MD: NIAAA, 2002).

Health Resources and Services Administration (HRSA), *Changing Demographics: Implications for Physicians, Nurses and Other Health Workers*, (Rockville, MD: DHHS, 2003), *Online,* <http://bhpr.hrsa.gov /healthworkforce/reports/changedemo/Content.htm>, Oct. 2004.

Heathfield, S.M., "Ten Tips to Make Training Work," 2004, *Online,* <http://humanresources.about.com/library/weekly/aa081400a.htm>, Oct. 2004.

Institute of Medicine (IOM), Committee on the Health Professions Education Summit, *Health Professions Education: A Bridge to Quality,* (Washington, DC: National Academy Press, 2003).

Institute of Medicine (IOM), *Crossing the Quality Chasm: A New Health System for the 21st Century,* (Washington, DC: National Academy Press, 2001).

Institute of Medicine (IOM), *In the Nation's Compelling Interest: Ensuring Diversity in the Health Care Workforce*, (Washington, DC: National Academy Press, 2004).

Institute of Medicine (IOM), *Managing Managed Care: Quality Improvements in Behavioral Health*, (Washington, DC: National Academy Press, 1997).

Isaacson, J.H., M. Fleming, M. Kraus, R. Kahn and M. Mundt, "A National Survey of Training in Substance Use Disorders in Residency Programs," *Journal of Studies on Alcohol* 61(6), 2000, pp. 912-915.

Jamieson, A., A. Curry and G. Martinez, "School Enrollment-Social and Economic Characteristics of Students," *Current Population Reports,* (Washington, DC: U.S. Census Bureau, 2001).

Johnson & Johnson, "Johnson & Johnson Helping to Reduce Nursing Shortage Enrollment: Rates Up at Nursing Schools Nationwide/More Funding for Nursing Scholarships and Grants," *Johnson & Johnson News*, 2003, *Online*, <http://www.jnj.com/news/jnj_news/20030429_093808.htm>, Oct. 2004.

Kaplan, L., *Substance Abuse Treatment Workforce Environmental Scan,* (Washington, DC: Abt Associates Inc., 2003).

Kauffman, J.F. and G.E. Woody, "Matching Treatment to Patient Needs in Opioid Substitution Therapy," *Treatment Improvement Protocol (TIP) Series 20,* (Rockville, MD: SAMHSA/CSAT, 1995).

Knudsen, J. and R. Gabriel, *Advancing the Current State of Addictions Treatment: A Regional Needs Assessment of Substance Abuse Treatment Professionals in the Pacific Northwest,* (Portland, OR: RMC Research Corporation, 2003).

Knudsen, H.K., J.A. Johnson and P.M. Roman, "Retaining Counseling Staff at Substance Abuse Treatment Centers: Effects of Management Practices," *Journal of Substance Abuse Treatment* 24(2), 2003, pp. 129-135.

Landis, R., B. Earp and S. Libretto, *Report on the State of the Substance Abuse Treatment Workforce in 2002: Priorities and Possibilities*, (Silver Spring, MD: Danya International, Inc., 2002 Draft).

Levin, A., "IOM Report: Building a More Diverse Health Care Workforce," *Health Behavior Information Transfer (HABIT)* 7(2), 2004, *Online*, <http://www.cfah.org/habit/vol7no2/IOM report.cfm>, March 2005.

The Lewin Group, Inc., *The Clinical Workforce in the Substance Abuse Treatment System,* (Rockville, MD: DHHS, SAMHSA, 2004).

Lewin-VHI, Inc., *Substance Abuse Training Needs Analysis, Final Report*, (Alexandria, VA: The Lewin Group, Inc., 1994).

Marrelli, A., M. Hoge and J. Tondora, *Strategies for Competency Modeling*, (Rockville, MD: SAMHSA, 2004 Draft).

McCarty, D., "The Alcohol and Drug Abuse Treatment Workforce," *Frontlines: Linking Alcohol Services Research and Practice,* (Bethesda, MD: NIAAA, 2002).

McLellan, A.T., D. Carise and H. Kleber, "Can the National Addictions Treatment Infrastructure Support the Public's Demand for Quality Care?" *Journal of Substance Abuse Treatment* 25(2), 2003, pp. 117-121.

McLellan, A.T., "Privacy and Substance Abuse Issues," *Hearings on Privacy and Health Information Technology,* (Washington, DC: NCVHS, 2005), *Online*, <http://www.ncvhs.hhs.gov/050223ag.htm>, March 2005.

Meier, P.S., C. Barrowclough, and M.C. Donmall, "The Role of the Therapeutic Alliance in the Treatment of Substance Misuse: A Critical Review of the Literature," *Addictions* 100(3), 2005, pp. 304-316.

National Association for Addiction Professionals (NAADAC), *The Association for Addiction Professionals' Year Two Final Report: A Survey of Early Career Substance Abuse Counselors*, (Alexandria, VA: NAADAC, 2003).

National Association of Social Workers Practice Research Network (NASW PRN), "Informing Research and Policy Through Social Work Practice," *NASW PRN Survey Final Report,* (Rockville, MD: CSAT, 2001).

National Association of State Alcohol and Drug Abuse Directors (NASADAD), *Recommendations Related to Closing the Treatment Gap,* NASADAD Policy Position Paper, 2003.

Nevidjon, B. and J. Erickson, "The Nursing Shortage: Solutions for the Short and Long Term," *Online Journal of Issues in Nursing,* 2001, *Online*, <http://www.nursingworld.org/ojin/topic14/tpc 4.htm>, June 2004.

New Freedom Commission on Mental Health, *Achieving the Promise: Transforming Mental Health Care in America, Final Report,* (Rockville, MD: DHHS, SAMHSA, 2003).

Office of Alcoholism and Substance Abuse Services (OASAS), *The Addictions Profession: A Workforce in Crisis, A Compilation of the Results of the 2001 Regional Workforce Development Focus Groups*, (Albany, NY: NYS OASAS, 2002).

Roy-Byrne, P., "Therapeutic Alliance and Psychotherapy Outcome," *Journal Watch for Psychiatry*, 1996, *Online*, <http://psychiatry.jwatch.org /cgi/content/full/1996/901/1>, April 2005.

Saitz, R., K. Mulvey and A. Plough, "Physician Unawareness of Serious Substance Abuse," *American Journal of Drug and Alcohol Abuse* 23(3), 1997, pp. 343-354.

Scanlon, W.J., "Nursing Workforce: Recruitment and Retention of Nurses and Nurse Aides Is a Growing Concern," *GAO testimony,* (Washington, DC: GAO, 2001), *Online,* <http://www.gao.gov/new.items/d01750t.pdf>, Oct. 2004.

Stoffelmayr, B.E., B.E. Mavis, L.A. Sherry and C.W. Chiu, "The Influence of Recovery Status and Education on Addiction Counselors' Approach to Treatment," *Journal of Psychoactive Drugs* 31(2), 1999, pp. 121-127.

Substance Abuse and Mental Health Services Administration/Center for Substance Abuse Treatment (SAMHSA/CSAT), "Addictions Counseling Competencies: The Knowledge, Skills and Attitudes of Professional Practice," *Technical Assistance Publication (TAP) Series 21,* (Rockville, MD: DHHS, 2002).

Substance Abuse and Mental Health Services Administration (SAMHSA), *Trends in Substance Abuse Treatment Admissions: 1992-2000 Treatment*

Episodes Data Set (TEDS), (Rockville, MD: DHHS, 2002), *Online*, <http://wwwdasis.samhsa.gov/teds00/TEDS 2K Chp2.htm>, Oct. 2004.

Substance Abuse and Mental Health Services Administration (SAMHSA), *A National Review of State Alcohol and Drug Treatment Programs and Certification Standards for Counselors and Prevention Professionals*, (Rockville, MD: DHHS, 2005).

Sullivan, S., "Wellness Programs," *e-HResources.com,* 2000, *Online,* <http://www.ehresources.com/Articles/Nov2.htm>, Nov. 2000.

Taleff, M.J., "The State of Addictions Education Programs: Results of a National Cross-Sectional Survey," *Journal of Teaching in the Addictions* 2(1), 2003, pp. 59-70.

U.S. Department of Labor, Bureau of Labor Statistics (BLS), *2002-2003 Occupational Outlook Handbook,* (Washington, DC: BLS, 2003).

III. SUMMARY

This report summarizes trends in addictions treatment and the challenges that confront the treatment workforce. Importantly, the report also articulates a vision for the treatment and recovery support workforce by presenting a series of recommendations aimed at strengthening the field's professional identity. The recommendations in this report reflect some of the best thinking in the field and are intended to provide momentum for ongoing discussions among stakeholders about specific implementation strategies. The recommendations also set the stage for concerted action by DHHS Operating Divisions, the ATTCs, States, national trade associations, credentialing and licensing bodies, and academic institutions. They offer an agenda for the addictions treatment field now and into the future.

Fundamental improvements in the conditions of the workforce will require the collective action of institutional and organizational partnerships in the public and private sectors. The effectiveness of the addictions treatment workforce rests on its ability to invest intelligently in its future, by developing systems to address issues of recruitment, retention and staff development. Other health care professions (e.g., nurses and physicians) have demonstrated that such efforts can prove effective. It is time that the addictions treatment field, in partnership with States and the Federal government follow that example, taking the steps necessary to address the challenges faced by the addictions treatment workforce. Only by doing this will the barriers to treatment access be addressed and the quality of care substantially improved.

IV. Participants

This section acknowledges the participants who gave their time and input at a series of stakeholder meetings and contributed many of the ideas and recommendations included in this report. The listing of participants and their organizations on this roster does not imply organizational endorsement of this report. Careful efforts have been made to ensure that all stakeholders who contributed to the development of this report are recognized and listed. Any omissions or exclusions are unintentional.

I. Key Leaders Meeting: January 15, 2004

Jacqueline Butler, M.S.W., LISW, CCDC
Professor of Clinical Psychiatry
University of Cincinnati
College of Medicine, Substance Abuse Division
Cincinnati, OH

Eldon Edmundson, Ph.D.
Associate Professor
Department of Public Health & Preventive Medicine
School of Medicine
Oregon Health & Science University
Portland, OR

Heinrich Harwood
Vice President
The Lewin Group, Inc.
Falls Church, VA

Jerome Jaffe, M.D.
Clinical Professor
University of Maryland
Columbia, MD

Constance Pechura, Ph.D.
Senior Program Officer
The Robert Wood Johnson Foundation Princeton, NJ

Paul Roman, Ph.D.
Distinguished Research Professor of Sociology and
Director
Center for Research on Behavioral Health and
Human Services
University of Georgia
Athens, GA

Angela Warner
Executive Director
Institute for Professional Development in the
Addictions (IPDA)
Albany, NY

II. Trade Association Leaders Meeting: February 12, 2004

David Bergman
Director of Legal and Government Affairs
American Association for Marriage and Family Therapy
Alexandria, VA

John J. Coppola
President-Elect
State Associations of Addiction Services
Albany, NY

Michael Couty, M.A.
Director
Division of Alcohol and Drug Abuse
Department of Mental Health
Jefferson City, MO

Linda Hay Crawford
Executive Director
Therapeutic Communities of America
Washington, DC

Roger A. Curtiss, NCACII, LAC
President
The Association for Addiction Professionals
Alexandria, VA

Elaine Feeney
Awards Committee Chair
International Nurses Society on Addictions
Raleigh, NC

Pat Ford-Roegner, M.S.W., RN, FAAN
Executive Director
The Association for Addiction Professionals
Alexandria, VA

Lewis E. Gallant, Ph.D.
Executive Director
National Association of State Alcohol and Drug
Abuse Directors (NASADAD)
Washington, DC

Michael Harle
President/Executive Director
Gaudenzia, Inc. Norristown, PA

Laura Horton, Ed.D.
Vice President
International Certification & Reciprocity
Consortium/Alcohol and Other Drug Abuse
Indianapolis, IN

David Kaplan, Ph.D.
Associate Executive Director
American Counseling Association
Alexandria, VA

Marianne T. Marcus, Ed.D., RN, FAAN
Associate Fellowship Director
HRSA-AMERSA-SAMHSA/CSAT Fellowship

University of Texas – Houston
Houston, TX

Eileen McGrath, J.D.
Executive Vice President/Chief Executive Officer
American Society of Addiction Medicine
Chevy Chase, MD

Michael P. Melendez, LICSW, BCD
Training Director
Association for Medical Education and
Research in Substance Abuse
Simmons College School of Social Work
Boston, MA

Mark W. Parrino
President
American Association for the Treatment of
Opioid Dependence
New York, NY

Howard B. Shapiro, Ph.D.
Executive Director
State Associations of Addiction Services
Washington, DC

Mickey J.W. Smith, M.S.W.
Senior Policy Associate for Behavioral Health
National Association of Social Workers
Washington, DC

Angie Wainwright
Associate Director
International Certification & Reciprocity
Consortium/Alcohol and Other Drug Abuse
Falls Church, VA

III. Great Lakes Region Meeting: March 1, 2004

Lonnetta Albright
Director
Great Lakes Addiction Technology Transfer Center
Jane Addams College of Social Work
University of Illinois at Chicago
Chicago, IL

Tom Cox
Executive Director
Amethyst House
Bloomington, IN

Mike Florek
Chief Executive Officer
Tellurian Unified Community Addictions Network
(UCAN), Inc.
Monona, WI

Judith Glenz
Executive Director
Jackie Nitschke Center, Inc.
Green Bay, WI

Oren Hammes, MSSW, LCSW
Clinical & Criminal Justice Coordinator
WI Department of Health & Family Services
Madison, WI
Deborah Hollis
Director
Division of Substance Abuse Quality & Planning
Department of Community Health
Bureau of Mental Health & Substance Abuse Services
Lansing, MI

Sarah Moscato
Acting Chief Executive Officer
Illinois Alcoholism and Drug Dependence

Association
Springfield, IL

Colleen O'Donnell, M.S.W.
Project Manager
National Association of State Alcohol & Drug Abuse
Directors (NASADAD)
Washington, DC

Sam Price
Executive Director
Ten-Sixteen Treatment Centers
Midland, MI

Michael Reagan
President
Association of Licensed Substance Abuse
Treatment Professionals
Lansing, MI

Sally Reams
Administrator
Michiana Addictions and Prevention
Services
Three Rivers, MI

Sanford Starr
Chief
Planning, Outcomes and Research
Department of Alcohol & Drug Addictions Services
Columbus, OH

Lee Strawhun
President
Southlake Center for Mental Health
Merrillville, IN
Eloise Traina
Executive Director
Family Recovery Center Lisbon, OH

Rick Velasquez
Executive Director
Youth Outreach Services, Inc.
Chicago, IL

John Viernes
Deputy Director
Division of Mental Health, Family & Social Services
Administration
Indianapolis, IN

Theodore Ziegler
Chief Executive Officer
Community Health Center
Akron, OH

IV. Colleges and Universities Meeting: March 18, 2004

Mark Ala,
LMFT Part-Time Faculty
Saddleback Community College
Mission Viejo, CA

Amanda Baker
Coordinator of External Relations
Center for the Study of Addictions
Texas Tech University
Lubbock, TX

Joseph D. Biscoe III
Assistant Professor
Northwestern State University
Natchitoches, LA

Kirk Bowden
Chair
Chemical Dependency Program
Rio Salado College

Tempe, AZ

Eldon Edmundson, Ph.D.
Associate Professor
Department of Public Health & Preventive Medicine
School of Medicine
Oregon Health & Science University
Portland, OR

Ric Evans, M.A.
Director of Therapy, Adjunct Instructor
Division of Social Science
Kansas City Kansas Community College
Kansas City, KS

John T. Franklin, Ph.D.
Professor and Chair
Department of Counseling and Addictions Studies
University of Detroit Mercy
Detroit, MI

Anne S. Hatcher
Director
Center for Addictions Studies
Metropolitan State College, Denver
Denver, CO

Constance M. Horgan, Ph.D.
Professor and Director
Schneider Center for Behavioral Health
Brandeis University
Heller School for Social Policy and Management
Waltham, MA

Brian McCabe, M.S.W.
Coordinator
Chemical Dependency Program
Hudson Valley Community Center
Troy, NY

Robert J. Reid, Ph.D.
Assistant Professor
School of Social Work
Rutgers University
New Brunswick, NJ

Nancy A. Roget
Principal Investigator
Project Director
Mountain West Addiction Technolgy Transfer Center
(ATTC)
Reno, NV

David Schreiber
Addictions Counseling Instructor
Minneapolis Community and Technical College
Minneapolis, MN

Anne Helene Skinstad, Ph.D.
Assistant Professor
University of Iowa
College of Public Health
Department of Community Behavioral Health
Iowa City, IA

Susan A. Storti, Ph.D., RN
Research Associate/PI
Brown University
Center for Alcohol and Addictions Studies
Providence, RI

Michael Taleff, Ph.D., CSAC, MAC
Coordinator
Center for Substance Abuse
University of Hawaii
Honolulu, HI

V. Mid-America/Gulf Coast Region Meeting: March 24, 2004

Joseph D. Biscoe III
Assistant Professor
Northwestern State University
Natchitoches, LA

Patrick Clancey
Executive
The Patrician Movement
San Antonio, TX

David Coleman
Corporation Supervisor
Wilbur Mills Center
Searcy, AR

Michael Duffy
Assistant Secretary
Office of Addictive Disorders
Department of Health & Hospitals
Baton Rouge, LA

Janice Fox
Administrator
Acadiana Recovery Center
Lafayette, LA

M. Trost Friedler
Executive Director
Harbor House Recovery Center
Jackson, MS

Jennifer Glover, M.S., LPC
Clinical Treatment Services Coordinator
Substance Abuse Services
Oklahoma City, OK

Joe M. Hill
Director of Alcohol and Drug Abuse Prevention
Department of Human Services
Division of Behavioral Health Services
Little Rock, AR

Cynthia Humphrey
Executive Director
Association of Substance Abuse Programs
Kerrville, TX

Herbert Loving
Director
Division of Alcohol & Drug Abuse
Department of Mental Health
Jackson, MS

Colleen O'Donnell
Project Manager
National Association of State Alcohol and Drug
Abuse Directors (NASADAD)
Washington, DC

Joyce O'Neal
Executive Director
Monarch, Inc.
Muskogee, OK

Jeff Smith
Assistant Director
Quapaw House Treatment Center
Hot Springs, AR

Richard Spence
Research Scientist
Gulf Coast Addiction Technolgy Transfer Center
(ATTC)
Center for Social Work Research
University of Texas

Austin, TX

Pat Stilen
Director
Mid-America Addiction Technolgy Transfer Center (ATTC)
Kansas City, MO

Marilyn Thoms
Director of Clinical Programs
Gateway to Prevention and Recovery
Shawnee, OK

David R. Wanser, Ph.D.
Executive Director
Texas Commission on Alcohol & Drug Abuse Austin, TX

VI. Federal Agencies Meeting: April 8, 2004

Donna M. Bush
Drug Testing Team Leader
Center for Substance Abuse Prevention, SAMHSA
Rockville, MD

Peggy A. Clark, M.S.W., MPA
Technical Director
Center for Medicaid and State Operations, Centers for Medicare and Medicaid Services
Baltimore, MD

Jennifer B. Columbel
Senior Policy Advisor for Substance Abuse
Bureau of Justice Assistance, Office of Justice Programs
U.S. Department of Justice
Washington, DC

Charles Gould
Manager

U.S. Navy Drug and Alcohol Program
U.S. Navy Bureau of Medicine and Surgery Washington, DC
Ronald Manderscheid, Ph.D. Chief, SAB, CMS
Center for Mental Health Services SAMHSA
Rockville, MD

Cruz Martinez
Substance Abuse Specialist
U.S. Department of Defense, Marine Corps
Quantico, VA

Christopher J. McLaughlin
Public Health Analyst
Health Resources and Services Administration
Bureau of Health Professions
Rockville, MD

Harold Perl, Ph.D.
Chief, Health Services Research Branch
National Institute on Alcohol Abuse and Alcoholism (NIAAA)
National Institutes of Health
U.S. Department of Health and Human Services
Bethesda, MD

Suman Rao, Ph.D.
Deputy Research Training Coordinator
National Institute on Drug Abuse
Bethesda, MD

Marcia M. Starbecker
Program Officer
Health Resources and Services Administration
Bureau of Health Professions
Division of State, Community and Public Health
Rockville, MD

Jack Stein, Ph.D.
Branch Chief

Services Research Branch
National Institute on Drug Abuse
Bethesda, MD

Richard T. Suchinsky, M.D.
Associate Chief for Addictive Disorders
Department of Veterans Affairs Washington, DC

Jim Swart
Acting Director
Office of Drug and Alcohol Policy and Compliance
U.S. Department of Transportation
Washington, DC

Helen S. Thornton, Ph.D.
Education Research Analyst
U.S. Department of Education
Office of Special Education and Rehabilitative Services
Washington, DC

Gregg Weltz
Program Manager
Office of Youth Services
U.S. Department of Labor
Washington, DC

VII. Human Resources Meeting: May 4, 2004

Mildred Brooke
Chief Executive Officer
Health Management Consultants
Columbia, MD

Andrew Buckner
Operations Manager Buffalo Valley
Hohenwald, TN

Judie Jobe
Vice President Human Resources Rosecrance, Inc.
Rockford, IL

Brenda McDonald
Human Resources Director
Michiana Addictions and Prevention Services
(M.A.P.S.)
Kalamazoo, MI

Michael Moyle, J.D.
Director of Fiscal and Corporate Operations Gaudenzia, Inc.
Norristown, PA

Richard Neubert
Executive Vice President
Operation PAR
St. Petersburg, FL

Bernardo Rodriguez
Vice President
Finance and Administration
VIP Services
Bronx, NY

Jose Soria
Deputy Director
Aliviane NO-AD, Inc.
El Paso, TX

Patricia Taylor
Director of Human Resources
Samaritan Village Jamaica, NY

Gina Trinidad
Director of Human Resources
Tarzana Treatment Center
Tarzana, CA

Eve Weinberg
Director of Human Resources and Training Treatment
Alternatives for Safe Communities (TASC)
Chicago, IL

VIII. Clinical Supervisors Meeting: May 19, 2004

William Bohannon, CCS, CADC
Clinical Supervisor
Wilbur Mills Substance Abuse Treatment Center
Searcy, AR

Alan Cook, M.A., LPC, LAC, MAC
Director
Cortez Addiction Recovery Services, Inc. (CARS)
Cortez, CO

Crescenzo De Luca
Assistant Director of Methadone Programs
Lower East Side Service Center
New York, NY

Jon Emerson
Program Manager
Cascadia Behavioral Healthcare
Hillsboro, OR

Karen Garrett, M.A., CAP, CAPP
Senior Director of Quality Improvement and Training
River Region Human Services
Jacksonville, FL

Susan Harris, CADC
Clinical Supervisor Thresholds, Inc.
Georgetown, DE

Earl Hill
Program Director

Western Psychiatric Institute and Clinic (WPIC)
Verona, PA

Paul Lauridsen
Clinical Director Stepping Stones
Joliet, IL

Michael S. Levy, Ph.D.
Director of Clinical Treatment Services
CAB Health & Recovery Services
Danvers, MA

Cathy Moonshine, Ph.D.
Director of Professional Services
De Paul Treatment Centers
Portland, OR

Margo Preston, CRADC
Program Coordinator
Lake County Health Department
Women's Residential Program
Vernon Hills, IL

David Wyman, BCSAC, BCAGC
Clinical Supervisor
Acadiana Recovery Center
Lafayette, LA

IX. Recovery Support Personnel Meeting: May 25, 2004

Sonya Baker
Project Manager
Community Recovery Network
Santa Barbara, CA

Mark Beresky
Co-Director
New England Alliance of Methadone Advocates

Brattleboro, VT

The Reverend J. David Else
Director
Center for Spirituality in 12 Step Recovery
Pittsburgh, PA

Sandra Gardner
Clinical Support Technician/Outreach Worker
Women at the Crossroads
Peoria, IL

Jean LaCour, Ph.D., CAPP
President
NET Training Institute
Orlando, FL

Cherie Hunter
Administrator
Restoring Citizenship
Treatment Alternatives for Safe Communities
(TASC)
Chicago, IL
Andre Johnson
Program Manager
The Detroit Recovery Project
Detroit, MI

Robert Savage
Project Director
Connecticut Community for Addictions Recovery
(CCAR)
Wethersfield, CT

Barbara Warren
Director of Organizational Development, Planning
and Research
SpeakOUT!: LGBT Voices for Recovery
New York, NY

David L. Whiters
Project Director
Recovery Consultants of Atlanta, Inc. Atlanta, GA

Jan Wrolstad
Associate Director
Mid-America Addiction Technolgy Transfer Center (ATTC)
Kansas City, MO

Center for Substance Abuse Treatment (CSAT) Staff

Mady Chalk, Ph.D.
Director
Division of Services Improvement
SAMHSA/CSAT
Rockville, MD

Kevin Chapman, D.Min.
Policy Assistant
Office of the Administrator SAMHSA
Rockville, MD
Donna M. Cotter, M.B.A.
Partners for Recovery Coordinator
Office of Program Analysis and Coordination
SAMHSA/CSAT
Rockville, MD

Karl D. White, Ed.D.
Public Health Analyst
Division of Services Improvement
SAMHSA/CSAT
Rockville, MD

Consultants

E. Lorraine Bell, R.N., JD, MPH
Senior Associate Abt Associates Inc.

Bethesda, MD

Peter Gaumond. M.A., L.S.W.
Senior Associate Abt Associates Inc.
Bethesda, MD

Margaret Gwaltney, M.B.A.
Senior Associate Abt Associates Inc.
Bethesda, MD

Linda Kaplan, M.A.
Chief Executive Officer
Global KL, LLC
Silver Spring, MD

Richard Landis, M.S.W.
President
Global KL, LLC
Silver Spring, MD

Melanie Whitter
Senior Associate
Abt Associates Inc.
Bethesda, MD

In: Strengthening …
Editor: Valentin LeBlanc
ISBN: 978-1-62808-683-6

Chapter 2

STRATEGIES FOR STRENGTHENING SUBSTANCE USE PREVENTION, TREATMENT, AND RECOVERY SYSTEMS: PROVIDER NETWORKS AND IMPACT ON THE WORKFORCE[*]

Joseph Hyde

NOTE: The authors don't work for the government.

EXECUTIVE SUMMARY

This study illustrates nine successful alcohol and other drug (AOD) addiction provider networks that are highly diverse in size, scope, complexity, and service array. These case studies are vignettes of the origins, current operations, strengths, and challenges of these networks. The reader will see how these organizations mounted strategies to address problems and challenges that are common throughout the addictions system.

The addictions treatment provider system is confronted with a variety of challenges in today's environment, including shrinking resources, increasing

[*] This report, dated January 2009, was released by the Substance Abuse and Mental Health Services Administration, Center for Substance Abuse Treatment, Partners for Recovery Initiative.

demands to demonstrate outcomes, patients with complex sets of problems calling for increased staff skills, and changes in business practices. These and other factors place high demands on the addictions treatment system. Small providers are especially hard-hit, unsure if they can continue to exist in this current environment, but large providers are not immune from the same struggles. Recruitment, retention, and professional development of staff are ongoing challenges to the field. Staff turnover rates in some areas are said to rival those in the fast-food industry (McLellan, Carise, and Kleber, 2003). To survive and grow, agencies must find new methods of collaborating in order to maximize resources, retain staff, find strength and stability in a changing marketplace, and provide higher quality services based on sound and appropriate evidence-based practices. In a report entitled "Strengthening Professional Identity: Challenges of the Addictions Treatment Workforce" (Whitter, Bell, Gaumond, and Gwaltney, et. al, 2006), it is recommended that network strategies be fostered in order to strengthen the infrastructure of agencies and sustain the workforce.

Although networks and collaboration are not new concepts, it is important to examine various types of collaborations for strategies and structures that can strengthen and support providers. Lessons that might be learned from these organizations may be replicated in other communities. Some of the challenges in one part of the country are truly not that different in other regions. This report provides a unique opportunity to look at how other communities brought solutions to these common problems.

BACKGROUND AND PURPOSE OF STUDY

The Substance Abuse and Mental Health Services Administration/Center for Substance Abuse Treatment (SAMHSA/CSAT) Partners for Recovery (PFR) initiative supported the development and implementation of this study of provider networks. It builds on recommendations from an earlier report entitled "Strengthening Professional Identity: Challenges of the Addictions Treatment Workforce" (Whitter, et. al., 2006). Within the Infrastructure section of the earlier report, recommendations were made to foster network development among substance use service providers. An excerpt from the report follows:

> As the addiction field faces agency closures, particularly among smaller treatment providers, networks represent an important mechanism

for ensuring agency viability and service availability. In addition, in some cases, networks can provide career paths for addiction professionals and potential staffing pools for member organizations.

In an effort to help strengthen management efficiency and ensure long-term sustainability, small addiction treatment providers may benefit from collaborative engagement in a network or use of a shared management organization to assist with human resource needs and clinical and administrative functions.

This sharing of resources results in economies of scale for participating agencies and also makes available critically needed supports, many of which would not be affordable otherwise to member agencies.

The current report is based on nine case studies of addictions provider networks and illustrates a range of collaborative approaches. Case studies cover a broad range of prevention and treatment agencies and networking strategies. The report describes

- a diversity of network structures, including networks that have become freestanding nonprofit organizations, networks where one organization is the administrative lead, and networks that are non-incorporated coalitions of providers;
- a diversity of collaboration, such as sharing staff, joint projects, shared management functions, and shared purchasing;
- a diversity of networking mechanisms, including joint funding, co-location, common client-tracking systems, and cross-training;
- a diversity of agreements, from negotiated contracts to "good faith" verbal agreements; and
- diverse scopes of service within networks, including both services to the community and services to network members.

Additionally, the report provides

- a demonstration of the value of networks,
- a discussion of strengths and challenges in networks, and
- a description by network members of considerations in founding networks.

Networks were selected for these case studies on the basis of diversity of collaborations, networking mechanisms and strategies, network agreements, and demonstrated effectiveness of networking. Networks were selected from across the country reflecting urban, suburban, and rural communities. Some selected networks had diverse populations, and others had targeted populations; some selected networks were composed of just a few agencies, and others were composed of many agencies.

The motivation for this report came from issues of workforce development in addictions systems. There have been numerous reports in recent years describing the workforce crisis in the field of addictions. The question has been raised, "What role can and do networks play in addressing workforce development?" At the time of network formation, workforce development ranked as a secondary issue for most of the networks surveyed. The two primary motivations for forming networks came from (1) very real concerns about the financial survival of community programs associated with sweeping changes in States such as the introduction of managed care and (2) a sincere commitment by providers and community leaders to build or strengthen capacity and build the workforce to provide quality services, including building capacity to provide recovery support services. As networks came together and became fully functioning, issues of workforce development came to play a more prominent role.

Project Approach and Methodology

Identification and Selection of Provider Networks

The State Associations of Addiction Services (SAAS) initially asked its member State provider associations to identify and submit names of potential networks for this report. Networks were loosely defined as collaborations between providers for the purpose of improving access to specialized services, expanding services, coordinating care, treating people with co-occurring mental or physical disorders, sharing staff, sharing information technology, sharing other administrative and management functions, co-locating staff or programs, achieving economies of scale, or enhancing revenue. These networks or collaborations could range from informal associations to highly organized and structured entities.

Nine criteria for the final selection of case studies were developed:

1. The network must consist of at least two separate cooperating agencies.

2. The network must have been operational for a period of time.
3. The network should assist in responding to workforce challenges.
4. At least one network member needs to be an organization whose primary function is providing addictions treatment.
5. At least one network must include member organizations that provides non-addictions-related services, such as housing and homeless, primary care, mental health, educational, vocational, or employment services.
6. At least one network should consist of only two agencies.
7. At least one network should be a large, formalized network that is separately incorporated or is based on memoranda of agreement that commit members to significant levels of collaboration, service coordination, and staff and/or resource sharing.
8. At least one network should serve minority or underserved populations (e.g., Native Americans, African-Americans, or homeless persons).
9. The selected networks should, to the extent feasible, be distributed geographically across the country.

The response to this initial request to the State provider associations identified 54 networks of various sizes and configurations involving as few as 2 agencies to as many as 50 and more agencies. Services provided within the networks were highly diverse. At the level of direct service, networks providing a full continuum of care were represented, and within the continuum of care an array of services was provided by traditional and nontraditional providers. In other networks, effective collaboration resulted in the operation of a single treatment program. The network selection reflected various degrees and types of infrastructure and a wide range of network membership services. For purposes of this project the decision was made that all networks had to be in operation for at least 5 years; one of the selected networks had been in operation for more than 40 years. SAAS received approval to conduct the case studies after submitting a preliminary selection of proposed networks to Abt Associates and CSAT under the PFR initiative.

Development of Interview Protocol

The next task in this project was to develop a standardized protocol for information to be collected. This protocol enabled more consistent collection of information across sites and comparisons of how different networks addressed core issues, and it guided telephone interviews and prompted collection of print and other information when available. In addition, public domain financial reports on nonprofits (Internal Revenue Service [IRS] Form 990), available through GuideStar (www.guidestar.org), were reviewed for a number of organizations.

Initial interviews were conducted during 2007, and follow-up contacts were made during the spring and summer of 2008. Case studies were drafted based on the data collected. These case studies are primarily descriptive and illustrate network operations. This report aims to provide options and illustrate real-world possibilities for networks that can strengthen the addictions infrastructure. Founders and operators of these networks are viewed as pioneers who took chances, worked very hard, and created sustained entities that have added value to their communities and to the lives of the persons they serve.

An effort was made to create a degree of uniformity within the case studies to make it easier to compare features across networks. Each case study addresses the following content areas:

• Organizational History • Mission, Values, and Vision • Network Structure • Membership • Geographic Area • Staffing • Range of Services	• Collaborative Efforts • Workforce Development • Strengths of the Network • Challenges of the Network • Considerations in Forming a Network • Looking to the Future

Nine Case Studies

Nine networks were chosen for case studies from nine different States. The networks are organized by State and shown below (see also the appendix for a summary of the networks, including Web site information when available):

- ***California—California Association of Addiction Recovery Resources (CAARR).*** CAARR is a large multiservice membership association providing training, technical assistance, legislative services, other membership services, and management oversight to several small nonprofit programs; hosting one of the State's counselor certification boards; and training and certifying "Sober Living Environments" (e.g., sober houses or recovery homes).

- ***Florida—Central Florida Behavioral Health Network (CFBHN).*** CFBHN is a management entity (Administrative Services Organization) operated by 19 mental health and substance use providers in nine counties in the Tampa Bay area and across central Florida managing and providing publicly funded behavioral health services to this region. Additionally, CFBHN coordinates county-based planning, training, and technical assistance to providers.
- ***Illinois—Project WIN (Wellness Initiative Network).*** Project WIN is a federally funded network of substance use and other service providers to address the needs of homeless adults with addiction and co-occurring disorders.
- ***Maine—Maine Juvenile Treatment Network (MJTN).*** MJTN is a network of providers supported through the Maine Office of Substance Abuse. This group of providers has developed unique sets of skills and evidence-based practices to treat the needs of adolescents with substance use disorders. The MJTN also serves as a statewide resource to support the screening and referral of youth into appropriate services.
- ***Massachusetts—Behavioral Health Services Network (BHSN).*** BHSN is a decentralized system of providers that includes private, not-for-profit agencies in the area providing supportive housing, substance use disorders treatment, and a range of community mental health services for persons with substance use and co-occurring disorders. The Somerville Mental Health Association serves as the lead agency for the network.
- ***Nebraska—Touchstone.*** Touchstone is an intensive residential treatment program serving adults with co-occurring disorders. The program was created and is operated by two collaborating agencies in Lincoln.
- ***New York—North Country Behavioral Healthcare Network (NCBHN).*** NCBHN, a rural behavioral health care network serving a large geographic region, provides an array of services for adults, adolescents, children, elderly people, and Native Americans. Through North Country Management Services (NCMS) the network also

provides a wide range of training, technical assistance, management support, and legislative liaison to its member agencies.

- ***North Carolina—Guilford County Substance Abuse Coalition (GCSAC).*** GCSAC is a coalition of organizations providing prevention and treatment services for substance use and mental health disorders. Members of GCSAC represent various sectors of the community, including hospitals, physicians, schools, law enforcement, local government, community organizations, and faith-based organizations.
- ***Oregon—Oregon Treatment Network (OTN).*** OTN is a network of providers for the treatment of substance use and co-occurring disorders. The network, which serves central Oregon, is part of the National Institute on Drug Abuse Clinical Trials Network.

Case Studies on Provider Networks by State

Case Study 1: California—California Association of Addiction Recovery Resources

Data Sources

- *Interview*: Susan Blacksher, Executive Director
- *Other sources*: printed materials, web-based materials, IRS Form 990 for 2006 and 2007

Organizational History

The California Association of Addiction Recovery Resources (CAARR), originally founded in 1972 as the California Association of Alcoholic Recovery Homes, is a 501(c)(3) membership organization with headquarters in Sacramento. CAARR was originally established as an association for recovery homes and has significantly expanded its size and scope of services since that time. Currently CAARR has over 150 member agencies, over 100 recovery homes, and a number of individual members; the association has an annual operating budget of approximately $1.5 million.

Members of the association subscribe to a social model of alcohol and other drug (AOD) recovery (California Department of Alcohol and Drug Programs, 2007). CAARR is a professional membership association, which also contracts with agencies to provide administrative services. The following services are provided by CAARR:

- Membership services
- Managing the statewide certification process to become a Certified Alcoholism and Other Addiction Specialist. Currently over 6,000 people are certified or in the process of becoming certified.
- Conducting statewide training and workforce development programs, including a year-long counselor training institute preparing persons in recovery to become certified as addictions treatment professionals. There is a regular schedule of training and continuing education programs.
- Conducting regional conferences
- Making technical assistance available to AOD programs statewide at no cost through a contract with the California Department of Alcohol and Drug Programs. Assistance is in the areas of program startup, executive coaching, policies and procedures development, program certification, program licensing, program design, board development, and fiscal management.
- Legislative monitoring and advocacy for AOD abuse programs and professionals
- Administrative management of recovery programs that lack sufficient business capacity to be self sustaining

CAARR is supported through a variety of grants and contracts that make up approximately 70 percent of the total revenue. The remaining income is based largely of member fees.

In 2000, CAARR expanded its scope of work beyond training, technical assistance, and advocacy to include administrative management of small recovery-oriented programs. This was originally done on a 1-year (trial) contract with a single small residential program on the verge of closure. CAARR now provides administrative management for four small programs, allowing these programs that would have otherwise closed to continue and prosper. It currently administers two of these programs while the other two are now successfully operating on their own.

Mission, Values, and Vision

The mission of CAARR is to encourage the development, expansion, and continuing quality of social model programs in California through advocacy, education, training, and positive role modeling.

The *social model* has been broadly described as a sociocultural model like Alcoholics Anonymous (AA). Those who subscribe to the social model believe that addiction is a multifaceted disease, one that is caused by a combination of factors: spiritual, biological, psychological, and social/environmental. Treatment and recovery are defined in relation to the person, community, and/or program, as compared to a traditional medical model that stresses the doctor-patient relationship. The model promotes the respect and dignity of the individual while also promoting personal and social responsibility. Recovery is characterized as something beyond thoughts, feelings, and behaviors and includes a change in lifestyle, which could include changes in the family, peers, and other groups. Community involvement in support of recovery is valued.

Network Structure

CAARR is an incorporated 501(c)(3) nonprofit membership organization with more than 300 active members. The organization is led by a full-time executive director and is governed by an elected board of directors. The board of directors is comprised of 15 individuals, with 3 alternates, representing CAARR's statewide membership. The board of directors elects officers for the board. All board and officer seats have term limits. The board of directors meets five times each year, and a full membership meeting is held annually in March. Elections to the board of directors are held during the annual full membership meeting.

CAARR routinely assesses the needs of its members and, through its members, the perceived needs within the community. CAARR develops long-range strategic plans that are approved by the board and the membership.

Board Committees

The board maintains a number of standing and ad hoc committees in such areas as training and workforce development, legislative affairs, membership services, program standards, and counselor certification. There is also an executive committee.

Membership

The network is supported by three categories of membership: Program Members, Supportive Business Members, and Individual Members.

Program Members: Any California community-based, peer-group–oriented, alcoholism or alcoholism and drug recovery corporation, sole proprietor, or partnership is eligible to become a voting member. Dues for program membership are based on the program's annual budget. Program

Members represent the full continuum of services from prevention to treatment and recovery support services.

Supportive Business Members: These are businesses that support Program Member organizations and their efforts but may not be actively involved in the delivery of client services. Supportive Business Members are not voting members.

Individual Members: All individuals who have an interest in social model programs, prevention, and recovery and wish to support CAARR and its mission can apply for membership.

Geographic Area

CAARR provides services statewide.

Staffing

CAARR is a funded and staffed organization with a full-time executive director, three other full-time employees, several part-time employees, a large cohort of paid consultants and trainers, and significant volunteer efforts from CAARR membership. The organization also retains the services of a registered lobbyist to monitor legislation and to support advocacy efforts on behalf of the organization.

Range of Services

Membership Services

- *Technical assistance and support.* Technical assistance can address a range of direct service and management needs and can include training, onsite consultation, meeting or process facilitation, and product development. Technical assistance is accessed through a simple written request process. Technical assistance recipients may assume a portion of the expenses for the service.
- *Advocacy.* The network retains the services of a registered lobbyist, who monitors legislation that could affect members and supports advocacy efforts for the network with the State legislature.
- *Discounts on insurance programs and other resources.* Through group-purchasing capacity, the network offers discounts to members on a range of insurance products and other goods, materials, and services.
- *Discounts on training and education.* Members are given discounts on CAARRsponsored training events.

- *Formal and informal communication.* CAARR publishes an association newsletter and actively uses electronic systems to disseminate information to members. CAARR also maintains a membership bulletin board for announcements and job vacancies. The association supports and facilitates ongoing informal communication and networking among members at all levels of the organization.

Administrative Management

CAARR provides administrative management for a number of smaller programs. Under a written management agreement with CAARR, CAARR staff provide administrative and programmatic oversight, including fiduciary management, for these programs. These programs maintain their separate corporate status with active governing boards and benefit from reduced overhead expenses and some economies of scale due to being managed by a larger entity.

Initially, there were concerns regarding potential conflicts of interest from within CAARR due to having a membership association provide oversight of a program (even contractually). It was described as an important process for the board to openly discuss and debate this action in depth before the board of CAARR ultimately voted in favor. CAARR providing administrative services was ultimately viewed as a way for some smaller entities to continue operation with a degree of autonomy, preserving the culture of the organization.

Profitability is difficult to achieve and maintain in small freestanding residential programs operating without additional sources of funding and support. A fee-for-service payment system, which has become standard for behavioral health reform across the country, is usually not able to cover all costs that an agency incurs in the operation of a successful program. Access to other sources of funding has become necessary for program survival.

Consolidation of services and functions enhances financial viability of these small programs. For example, something as simple as bulk buying for groceries for combined agencies lowers costs to each agency. Other and more significant cost-savings measures include having one functional executive director serving all agencies, one finance director to perform fiscal operations, and shared clinical supervision. These savings are reinvested into the programs through enhanced direct service staffing and program activities. The CAARR executive director is proactive in "joining" the staffs by being routinely accessible and by attending staff and case conference meetings at the programs. CAARR also supports a number of team-building activities, including a level of transparency in decisionmaking and seeking active staff participation in planning and decisionmaking.

CAARR has made a commitment to professional growth and development of staff members working in these programs. All staff members are allowed to attend training (at no charge to the staff member) in support of staff member efforts to become certified. When staff members are ready to become certified, CAARR pays the fees for certification. For certified workers, continuing education is available at no charge.

Beyond expected business functions, as part of the administrative management activities CAARR works with organizations to develop enhanced organizational practices to make the programs more successful within the current marketplace. Strategies to reduce waiting lists and to fill empty beds more quickly are used to enhance cash flow. Planning efforts are undertaken to diversify funding streams. CAARR, working with the agencies, has been successful in obtaining additional contracts to support program operations.

This model of contracted management is described as being successful, in part, because special attention has been given to making sure the staff and boards of each of these small agencies remains actively involved in decisionmaking. All major decisions are subject to board discussion and, when necessary, approval. The success of these efforts has resulted in saving programs that without intervention would have closed and has increased the stature of CAARR in the State.

Technical Assistance

CAARR has a contract from the Single State Authority to provide consultation and technical assistance to nonprofit, community-based providers of substance use disorders services. Management and program consultation is available for existing programs and to build capacity for startup ventures.

Technical assistance is available to the provider community in the following areas:

- program startup, including needs assessment, feasibility, plans for capacity building and community mobilization;
- executive coaching;
- development of policies and procedures;
- program certification;
- program licensing;
- program design;
- development of programs and services for special populations;

- funding and development;
- boards of directors development; and
- fiscal management.

A smaller and more specific consultation contract managed by CAARR is for "peer review" services. Peer review activities are required on an annual basis by the Federal block grants for substance use programs receiving block grant dollars. CAARR recruits, trains, and coordinates the efforts of peer reviewers.

CAARR provides specific technical assistance and training under the California Disability Access Project to increase opportunities for, as well as the abilities of, people with physical, sensory, and cognitive disabilities to address their AODrelated problems by

- reducing attitudinal, architectural, programmatic, communication, and fiscal barriers to accessing appropriate treatment and recovery services for people with disabilities;
- enhancing the cultural and linguistic appropriateness of AOD treatment and recovery program services for people with disabilities;
- improving the quality, quantity, and outcomes of these services; and
- providing training and/or technical assistance to the State and local AOD agencies and disability agencies statewide.

Technical assistance services include program and policy development, disability awareness and sensitivity training, introduction to AOD for disability agencies, clinical approach/treatment protocol development for persons with disabilities, architectural surveys, resource development, community forums, and telephone consultation when appropriate. The Disability Access technical assistance project serves AOD prevention, treatment, and recovery service providers and organizations, as well as allied disability service providers statewide.

Collaborative Efforts

CAARR has distinguished itself in several highly innovative collaborative efforts. CAARR provides contracted administrative services for a number of small programs, including administrative oversight, clinical supervision, and fiscal management, while allowing these programs to remain programmatically distinct. This collaborative effort helps to reduce operating costs and enables these programs to continue to survive.

CAARR hosts a substance use counselor certification board, which also helps to reduce operating costs. Co-locating the board onsite with one of the major State training contractors seems to provide a level of positive synergy for both training and certification.

CAARR provides training, support, standards, and a collective voice for "Sober Living Environments" (SLEs), entities that in other parts of the country are called sober houses, recovery homes, or Oxford Houses. In other parts of the country these sober programs operate with little or no support, programmatic standards, or oversight.

Workforce Development

CAARR operates a number of major training and workforce development programs. Costs for these programs are substantially covered by State contracts, so training can be offered at little or no charge or are supported by individual tuition. These programs are described below.

CAARR Institute

The CAARR Institute, which is fully self-supported was created in 1978 to offer an alternative form of education for recovering people working in the AOD field. Many had found recovery through participation in AOD programs and then chose to work in programs providing peer leadership and experience. It was found that although these individuals might understand the process of recovery that worked for them, they might lack the technical skills and knowledge necessary to be effective serving others. These adult learners in early sobriety were often hesitant to return to a traditional classroom setting. The institute was established and designed to be offered in easily accessible locations, in a setting and approach that was more conducive to an adult learner audience. Instructors recruited to teach the curriculum also came with significant field experience and could share real-life experiences with their students. Today the institute curriculum is based on SAMHSA's TAP 21 "Addiction Counseling Competencies: The Knowledge, Skills, and Attitudes of Professional Practice" (CSAT, 2006). The CAARR Institute recruits and trains approximately 850 trainees annually; the trainees participate in a 46-part (270-hour) series that helps to prepare them to work as entry-level substance abuse counselors and to become certified as addiction professionals. This program is conducted in both Spanish and English.

CAARR Training Programs

CAARR has State contracts to provide an array of substance use disorders training programs. These courses are approved for continuing education credits and are provided at no cost to participants.

Continuing Education Courses

CAARR offers a range of continuing education courses statewide, under contract with the Single State Authority. They conduct 300 days of training annually.

Intensive Management Training

Intensive Management Training is an advanced curriculum taught by experienced program managers. It includes modules that address the basic principles of management as well as areas of management unique to AOD programs.

CAARR II, Advanced Alcohol and Drug Studies

This advanced practice training series addresses acquisition of advanced clinical skills and also addresses co-occurring health and mental health issues in addictions treatment.

CAARR International

At the request of recovery providers in neighboring Mexico, the CAARR training programs were translated, and bilingual CAARR training staff traveled to Mexico to initially provide instruction at the CAARR Instituto de Mexico to students and then complete a training of trainers. This training program is now self-sustaining and operated by recovery professionals in that country. A similar program was developed for representatives from Korea. Classes are conducted using the CAARR Institute materials in both Korea and Los Angeles.

CAARR Sober Living Institute

This training program targets the unique set of needs of persons or groups seeking to set up or operate an SLE (recovery home, sober house, Oxford House). The program defines an SLE and provides information on program siting, zoning laws, landlord/tenant laws, business types, business practices, recommended house policies and practices, good neighbor policies, and ethics, in addition to other content unique to AOD programs.

Special Training Initiatives

CAARR routinely receives discretionary contracts for specific training initiatives. Currently, "Trauma Informed Care" is being integrated into residential programs. In recent years, these initiatives have also included training and supporting providers adopting evidence-based practices.

Counselor Certification

CAARR hosts and supports one of the State counselor certification boards. The board is an independent entity. Hosting the certification board through the association helps to greatly reduce costs for counselor certification. With 6,000 persons currently certified through this board, the cost savings are many thousands of dollars annually to counselors and providers.

Outreach and Recruitment of Targeted Counselors

As part of a commitment to recruit, train, and support a more diverse workforce, CAARR has developed local resources and scholarships to provide counselor training and mentor African-Americans and persons who are deaf or hard of hearing. Each year funding is provided for 12 African American trainees and 7 deaf trainees.

Sober Living Environments

SLEs, sometimes called recovery houses, sober houses, or Oxford Houses, began in the mid-1970s and operate in nearly all States. In California, they are not subject to any licensing or oversight by the State. Many of the persons operating these houses are persons with strong ties to the 12-step recovery community. Concern for the care and safety of vulnerable persons in early recovery coupled with reports of abuses and misconduct in some of these programs has led organizations such as CAARR to create voluntary processes for an SLE to become registered with the association and agree to a set of standards and to make available training and support to SLE operators.

In 1993, CAARR developed minimum standards for SLEs based on input from community program providers and consumers. Standards were viewed as the first step in asking this emerging industry to regulate itself. The second step was to develop a process whereby programs can be recognized by their peers for establishing and meeting minimum standards and agreeing to abide by those basic standards.

CAARR has established a registration process for homes meeting the Sober Living Standards. In this process, a facility states that it meets the standards and declares that it will continue to abide by the standards. The process includes annual visits by peers from other SLEs, who review them to assure that the standards are maintained. SLEs are listed on the Member Homes Section of CAARR.

Strengths of the Network

- This organization began over 30 years ago as a membership association for residential recovery programs, and, while it has grown dramatically in size and scope to more than 300 members today, it remains faithful to its founding principles.
- The association supports multiple opportunities for general members and the governance board to discuss and decide on the future and direction of the organization. This includes allowing opportunities for board members to actively discuss and come to agreement on, at times, controversial issues.
- The association created categories of membership whereby affiliate or complementary organizations and individuals who were not necessarily recovery service providers were allowed to become CAARR members.
- The association provides a wide range of membership services, including technical assistance and support, legislative advocacy, group purchasing with resulting discounts on insurance programs and other goods and services, discounts on training and education, and support for formal and informal communication among members.
- The association is strategically positioned as an entity that is part of a vital infrastructure supporting the operations of community-based providers through the dissemination of information, monitoring state legislative processes affecting the industry, delivering training and technical assistance, recruiting and training entry-level workers, and credentialing part of the workforce.
- The association has diversified its scope of services and its funding base.
- The association operates multiple innovative training and workforce development programs, including a training institute for persons in recovery seeking to work in the field of addictions, large-scale statewide continuing education programs, programs that support the adoption of evidence-based treatment practices, programs that support a Spanish-speaking workforce, programs that provide addictions recovery support services for persons who experience a range of

physical and cognitive disabilities, and programs for supervisory and management training.

- The association hosts one of the State-recognized counselor certification boards. Through hosting the board, costs for certification are kept lower and savings are passed on to individuals and agencies.
- CAARR has taken a proactive approach to the proliferation of SLEs in California and in 1993 developed the first set of voluntary standards for SLEs. The association developed a voluntary registration process for SLEs whereby participating entities agreed to certain sets of standards.
- CAARR expanded administrative management capacity by assuming the administrative operations for four small programs. Through this effort they have been able to sustain these programs in the community, allowing them to maintain their separate programmatic identity while sharing management, thus reducing administrative, fiscal, and supervisory expenses and benefiting from economies of scale in purchasing. CAARR has also provided technical assistance for these programs to enhance practices and to diversify funding.

Challenges of the Network

- The single greatest challenge confronting the association relates to the financial crisis in the State of California. A number of the association contracts were reduced mid–contract year, resulting in fewer services to members.
- The association must navigate a number of highly complex matters where issues of "dual relationship" need to be carefully worked through. For example, the association assumed management of four small programs, supported the certification board, and took a proactive stance regarding standards for the SLEs and registration of SLEs.
- Careful succession planning is required to develop and replace successful managers and leaders.
- There are significant challenges associated with "Proposition 5" (California's Nonviolent Offender Rehabilitation Act) and other nonviolent drug use offender legislation that involve serving a greatly expanded criminal justice systems (CJ) client population. At the client service level, often these clients present with higher levels of antisocial and "criminogenic" personality and behavioral features, requiring modifications to program operations and causing real

concern about blending more hardened prison populations with nonprison populations. Further complicating the issue is that CJ clients are incentivized for admissions through being reimbursed at a higher per diem rate than community referrals; thus, the CJ clients will be admitted over the community referrals. The treatment gap for non-CJ clients appears to be widening. Inherent in this dilemma is a problem with systems capacity, particularly at the residential level. There is a shortage of residential service capacity perpetuated by the higher costs of opening and operating these programs and community opposition to residential programs, particularly those programs serving those with addictions and criminals.

Considerations in Forming a Network

The leadership was asked to describe what they viewed as important considerations in forming a network. They identified the following considerations:

- The organizations involved must be committed and solidly behind the mission and the implementation model for the program.
- It is important that the association have a mechanism that supports open and productive communication of these concerns. Issues that involve potential conflict of interest usually occur; if a program is going to provide a more complex array of services, then these issues must have a forum for discussion and consideration.

Measuring the success of an organization is based ultimately on how well it serves the needs of its membership and how well it responds to the needs of the community.

Looking to the Future

Initiatives on the horizon for the association include building on membership capacity to serve more diverse populations, including persons with co-occurring disorders; supporting providers in adopting evidence-based practices; and assisting Supportive Living Environment's initiatives to support women in treatment.

Case Study 2: Florida—Central Florida Behavioral Health Network

Data Sources

- *Interview*: Richard Brown, CEO, Agency for Community Treatment (ACTS), Tampa; Chair, Regional Council for Hillsborough County
- *Interview:* Linda McKinnon, CEO, Central Florida Behavioral Health Network
- *Interview*: Robert Rihn, President, Central Florida Behavioral Health Network and CEO of Tri-County Human Services, Lakeland
- *Interview*: Lucia Maxwell, Management Consultant
- *Other sources*: organizational documents and Web-based materials

Organizational History

The Central Florida Behavioral Health Network (CFBHN) is a not-for-profit 501(c)(3) community services network incorporated in 1997 initially as a collaboration of substance use providers. Today CFBHN is a management entity for 19 mental health and substance use providers in nine counties in the Tampa Bay area and across central Florida. Starting in 2005, an additional 275 faith- and community-based providers were funded through a Federal Access to Recovery (ATR) grant. Although the ATR grant was not renewed in the State of Florida beyond 2007, the impact of the grant is noteworthy for the organization's history and current development. In 2006, CFBHN and the Polk County Health Plan entered into a contract for the provision of behavioral services. The following counties are currently served by the network: Pinellas, Pasco, Hillsborough, Manatee, Sarasota and De Soto Counties, Polk, Highlands and Hardee.

Through the organization's members and other contracted entities, mental health and substance use disorders programs are provided for low-income and other populations determined to be at high risk of substance use and co-occurring disorders in central Florida. This network is best described as an Administrative Services Organization (ASO). The board of directors is composed of representatives of provider organizations and selected community members.

An ASO is defined as a contractual arrangement under which an independent organization handles the administration of claims, benefits, and other functions for an insured group or on behalf of a public entity, such as a State Medicaid program. While an ASO manages some levels of risk conducting business within a fixed administrative cost structure, it usually does not assume any medical risk of its own. Rather, the insured group or public entity assumes ultimate medical and financial risk for the covered population. Beyond this basic core definition, ASOs can take on a variety of forms and functions and perform a broad array of administrative and management services. Administrative functions often include planning; human resources management; provider enrollment; regulatory compliance; information systems; contract management; provider and member services; claims administration; and data reporting. An ASO might also conduct utilization management and prospective review or authorization for care services. In addition, it may provide retrospective review and case management and develop clinical guidelines and credentialing services. An ASO may perform other functions beyond those of traditional managed care, such as staffing, training, quality improvement initiatives, and other activities to support the workforce and community wellness and prevention services (National Health Law Program, 2006).

CFBHN is the lead organization in this region for contracting and purchasing of publicly funded mental health and substance use services, regional planning, cross-systems collaboration, care integration, and systems improvements and innovations. The network manages the distribution of State and Federal funds for treatment and prevention of mental health and substance use disorders in its targeted region. Overall, more than 35,000 adults and children receive treatment services each year through the network, and 77,000 youth and adults benefit from prevention services. Through its network of providers, a full array of treatment, early intervention, prevention, and recovery support services are provided, spanning all levels of care.

Mission, Values, and Vision

The goal of CFBHN is to provide well-managed and integrated behavioral health service delivery systems that increase access to care, improve continuity of care to vulnerable populations, prevent duplication of effort, reward efficiencies, and encourage exemplary practices within their regional geographic areas. This goal is to be accomplished through the network's guiding principles:

- To create a model for behavioral health and human service needs that embraces managed care concepts and is community based and client driven
- To be recognized as the community leader in providing behavioral health and other human services in the field

- To determine and promote best practices in services at the State and community levels
- To provide services for persons with mental health, addictions, and co-occurring disorders
- To maximize network capabilities through agency operability, emphasizing sharing of expertise in all administrative, clinical, automation, and management functions

Network Structure

Legal Structure

CFBHN is an incorporated 501(c)(3) nonprofit membership organization; currently it has 19 active member agencies and 5 community representatives. The member agencies span a nine-county geographic region covering approximately one-fourth of the State. The network is divided into four regions, each with its own elected regional chair and advisory committees. The regional councils are staffed by network staff, board members, and community stakeholders. These councils, which are permanent committees of CFBHN, meet monthly to plan for their areas, provide oversight into how providers are utilizing funds, look at outcomes, study different areas of service design that need further development, and recommend fund allocations.

Board members are elected and nominations are put forward to the network by a nominating process the board has developed. The bylaws require that member agency representatives account for 80 percent of the board's membership.

The board also has five public or community members through various community stakeholders than can include consumers. These five members are chosen by the board, which seeks to broaden its scope with these choices and also looks at maintaining good geographic distribution within the total area of CFBHN. Public funders require that public members or consumers serve on boards in order to receive grants. The public members in the past have included

- a local minister;
- a professor of business from a local university;
- a local president of a NAMI (National Alliance on Mental Illness) chapter;

- a professor of anthropology (who served on a substance abuse and mental health planning council and has a lengthy history with, and knowledge of, the service delivery system); and
- a former administrator from the State Juvenile Justice System.

The CFBHN board has an internally elected executive committee, which meets monthly. The full board meets at least six times per year. CFBHN has an active committee structure that includes an executive committee, a finance committee, a management information systems committee, a quality improvement committee, and it has member services, and the four regional councils. The network also has multiple ad hoc committees that are driven by current or emerging needs (e.g., co-occurring disorders, children's services).

The network also plays an active role in training and workforce development within the region, as discussed in a later section.

CFBHN's administrative office in Tampa maintains departments for program development, quality management, contracting, finance and accounting, billing, management information systems, purchasing and resource management functions, human resources, and provider services.

Regional Councils

The regional councils have expanded in scope over time and are now used for a number of different tasks. Meeting monthly, they provide oversight into how the providers are using their funds, monitor different areas of service design that need to occur, and provide assistance to agencies developing a business plan. The councils have played a central role in monitoring, planning, and recommending resource allocations. This has been accomplished by using performance measurements and benchmarking, assessing agency capacity to deliver services, and fully utilizing funds and ensuring contract compliance. Each regional council reviews all provider performance in their region on a monthly basis and has the capacity to recommend fund re-allocation. These recommended changes in fund allocation must be ratified by CFBHN's full board. Any re-allocation in excess of $50,000 requires the approval of the State contract office. Allocations less than $50,000 can be made internally within the network. In general, services to be covered are funded according to priorities established by the regional council planning, the State's gap analysis process, and the State plan for substance use and mental health services. Any new funding that becomes available to CFBHN is allocated to each county based on an agreed-upon equity formula unless it has been earmarked for a target population. Lastly, if no current network member can provide a specific service, the council can make and approve recommendations for new service providers.

CFBHN seeks to be inclusive outside its membership. Stakeholders and providers in the area who are not members are invited to participate in regional councils, quality improvement committees, and other meetings if there are agenda items of interest to those nonmembers.

Membership

There are currently 19 organizational members in the network representing a full range of addiction prevention, treatment, and recovery services and mental health/psychiatric services. To be a full network member, the organization must be a 501(c)(3) nonprofit holding contracts and necessary licenses with the State substance use and mental health program office, be an eligible Medicaid provider, have national accreditation by the Commission on Accreditation of Rehabilitation Facilities (CARF) or Joint Commission on Accreditation of Healthcare Organizations (JCAHO) (now the Joint Commission), and demonstrate financial stability and a commitment to the core principles and values of the network. Members enter into a contractual agreement joining CFBHN and agree to pay (nominal) annual dues as members. Other community providers participate in the network as contracted providers.

Geographic Area

The counties currently served by the network are Pinellas, Pasco, Hillsborough, Manatee, Sarasota and De Soto Counties, Polk, Highlands and Hardee.

Staffing

Currently, there are 22 full-time employees; consultants are hired as needed.

Range of Services

- *Provider network management*. This includes defining continuum of care and service array within the continuum; determining the types, number, and qualifications of providers based on community needs; selecting providers; credentialing; communication with providers; and training and technical assistance to providers.
- *Strategic planning for CFBHN.* This includes review of service data, utilization data, access, outcomes, and satisfaction; needs assessment;

gap analysis and provider input; setting measurable goals and objectives; and developing action plans and plans to monitor and evaluate.

- *Regional planning.* This planning is conducted through the regional councils and communicated to the full board.
- *Quality improvement / quality management.* The utilization management process includes definition of which services require prior approval, definition of "medical necessity," monitoring use of least restrictive levels of care, reviewing continued medical necessity, setting continued care criteria, and conducting retrospective review.
- *Utilization management.* The utilization management process defines which services require prior approval, definitions of "medical necessity," monitoring use of least restrictive levels of care, review of continued medical necessity, continued care criteria and retrospective reviews.
- *Financial management.* This includes regulatory compliance, proper accounting safeguards, analysis of clinical utilization and cost data, rate setting, claims processing, member services, and quality improvement activities and reporting.
- *Information management.* This includes client tracking, admissions, authorization, continued stay, integration of assessment and service planning data, supporting "seamless" transitions across levels of care, claims management, aggregate reporting, and outcomes and utilization analysis.
- *Provider services.* These services include business management technical assistance, clinical practice development (adoption of evidence-based practices), training, and education.

Collaborative Efforts

Through this collaborative entity regional service providers have come together to assume expanded responsibilities for community needs assessment, service planning, fund management, service delivery, and monitoring of outcomes for services to clients within their region. Access to services has been improved and coordination of efforts across programs has been enhanced through this collaboration. Because this administrative service entity is primarily organized around efficient service delivery and not as a profit center, the cost of managing public dollars is greatly reduced.

Workforce Development

CFBHN conducts a number of workforce development initiatives.

Quality Improvement / Evidence-Based Practices

The network, through its quality improvement processes, has made a commitment to supporting the adoption of evidence-based practices within the provider system. In recent years, this has included all CFBHN members that have co-occurring disorders capability with a strong emphasis on "systems of care" development and recovery-oriented systems. Systems of care is an approach to services that recognizes the importance of family, school, and community and seeks to promote the full potential of every child and youth by addressing their physical, emotional, intellectual, cultural, and social needs (http://www.systemsofcare.samhsa.gov/). Recovery-oriented systems support person-centered and self-directed approaches to care that build on the strengths and resilience of individuals, families, and communities to take responsibility for their sustained health, wellness, and recovery from alcohol and drug problems (CSAT, 2005).

Clinical Supervision

The role of clinical supervision in providing quality care and staff growth and development has been well recognized, but it has suffered significantly within the highly managed fee-for-service environment of most systems. CFBHN, through advocacy, has been successful in obtaining reimbursement for clinical supervision.

Training

CFBHN has received the appropriate designation required to offer Continuing Education Units for licensed clinicians. The network is able to share training opportunities across the system, resulting in savings to providers, shared knowledge, and collegial networking and support among practitioners. The network has also developed some online course capacity.

Increased Negotiating Power

The advocacy of the network has allowed CFBHN to obtain reimbursement rates for substance use disorders services moving toward parity with mental health services rate structures.

Sharing of Staff

CFBHN has facilitated staff sharing and co-location. Staff from different provider agencies have been co-located to provide services with other agency programs. Agencies have come together to share a physician staff position, which helps cut costs at each agency. Two agencies also shared a bond issue and purchased a building together.

Technical Assistance

CFBHN has provided significant assistance in working with agencies to develop information technology (IT) systems and provide assistance to new member management staff that were unfamiliar with management and responsibility for public mental health and substance use disorders funds managed through the network.

Administrative Process

CFBHN has been the recipient of a NIATx STAR-SI (Strengthening Treatment Access and Retention-State Implementation) grant for treatment improvement. This is an infrastructure cooperative agreement program that promotes systems-level implementation of process improvement methods to improve access to and retention in treatment (https://www.niatx.net). In the first year of that grant, two of the network's providers participated; they have now become mentors/leaders for other providers in the network that choose to participate. Not only was the NIATx model used for treatment improvement with providers, but CFBHN was able to use NIATx principles to improve internal administrative process for their staff.

Strengths of the Network

- The 19 member agencies are all committed to the success of the network and to changing the way behavioral health care is planned, administered, and implemented, consistent with a data-driven and consumer-focused planning process.
- The administrative costs for operating the network are low—approximately 5 percent in fiscal year (FY) 2007. This rate is dramatically lower than administrative costs commonly associated with managed care organizations (MCO).
- As the management entity for multiple streams of funding, the organization has the unique capability to braid and blend public dollars in order to create unique service arrays for persons served. It also helps to reduce overhead and unnecessary duplication.

- There is a commitment to operationalizing systems of care and recovery-oriented systems of care principles and values within the network.
- The network maintains a high-quality professional staff.
- Network staff demonstrate a high level of membership service (customer service).
- The network has the capacity to facilitate collaborative ventures among members.
- The network provides multiple venues for members and the community to provide formal and informal input into needs assessment and planning processes. The regional councils are inclusive of community stakeholders.
- The network has developed a highly sophisticated management information system.
- The network has achieved the highest levels of outcomes in the State. They have served more people than anywhere else in the State, with the highest outcomes for treatment success, and they have lowered wait list times.
- The network has developed sufficient infrastructure and capacity to compete successfully with any managed care or health maintenance organization in the State and at a much lower operating cost.
- The network has improved continuity of care.
- The network allows economies of scale that result in lowered administrative costs and maximization of resources to serve clients.
- The network administers Federal and State funds through a provider-operated system rather than a government entity or a traditional MCO. This demonstrates to State government and to private funders that a private, not-for-profit entity of provider-sponsored networks can offer a standard method of administering services to those with substance use and mental health disorders.
- The network hosts providers across the continuum of behavioral health care and primary health care. These providers include primary care hospitals, health centers, mental health facilities, and substance use disorders facilities (including both inpatient and outpatient); prevention agencies; and agencies with an emphasis on domestic violence and criminal justice services.

This network has created a platform for representatives from multiple agencies to sit together at both the regional planning council level and at the full network board level; this greatly benefits clients by enhancing coordination of services and reducing service silos. It is known from both experience and the data that in many cases these clients use the services of more than one member agency.

Challenges of the Network

- The high level of oversight and reporting to funders is a challenge. This has resulted in what has been describes as "meticulous" financial monitoring and safeguards that are labor intensive.
- The initial network had been greeted with a degree of caution as public dollars were distributed through a network to providers who control the actions and direction of the network. The performance of the organization over the past decade has reduced much of this caution.
- A major obstacle to beginning a network is the lack of a sophisticated IT infrastructure. Lack of an IT system severely limits the amount and types of data on clients, funding streams, and other information necessary for operating a successful program.

Considerations in Forming a Network

The leadership of CFBHN was asked to describe what they viewed as important considerations in forming a network. They identified the following considerations:

- Developing successful IT systems is a necessary capital expense.
- Regularly assess needs of your members and of the communities you serve.
- Commit to quality improvement processes.
- Clearly define your vision for the organization based on a commitment of services to the community.

Looking to the Future

Despite the loss of ATR funds to the State of Florida, there have been important lessons learned by the network that efforts are being made to sustain. These include the use of a Web-based voucher system where consumers of service exercise greater control over location of services, use of nontraditional recovery support providers, and use of recovery coaches. Preliminary data showed that the use of recovery coaches was highly instrumental in reducing or eliminating the need for longer term residential care in a number of cases. The network is in discussion with the University of South Florida to participate in a research study project to look in depth at some of these outcomes.

Recent changes in the State will result in the opportunity for Community Mental Health Services Block Grant (MHBG) funds to be managed through an ASO or MCO. The network is preparing for the opportunity to compete for these funds in their service region. The management entity structure developed by CFBHN is becoming the model for the State.

Case Study 3: Illinois—Project WIN

Data Sources

- *Interview*: Terry Johnson, Vice President and Chief Clinical Officer, South Suburban Council on Alcoholism and Substance Abuse, Chicago
- *Other sources*: organizational documents and Web-based materials

Organizational History

Project WIN (Wellness Initiative Network) was created as the result of grant funds provided by the U.S. Department of Housing and Urban Development (HUD) to the Cook County Department of Public Health (CCDPH) of Illinois. The Federal funding was to support the provision of a wide array of services to a targeted population of homeless adults in the southern and western part of the metropolitan Chicago / Cook County area. Project WIN became the collaborative work of eight agencies in the metropolitan Chicago area. CCDPH functions as the lead (and fiduciary) agent for Project WIN, and the participating agencies operate within the program through written partnership agreements. CCDPH provides most of the staff and administrative functions, receives all the funds, channels those funds in accordance with the agreements to the various agencies supplying services, receives all the reports from those agencies, and reports to HUD. Overall, the agencies see more than 400 homeless persons annually through Project WIN.

Project WIN is a multiagency, multiservice collaboration to provide coordinated care in the areas of mental health, medical health, and substance use treatment and housing to homeless adults. To engage homeless persons in these critical services, a team of clinicians provides active outreach and onsite services to clients. The network provides an expanded and coordinated array of services for a target population.

Mission, Values, and Vision

Project WIN is designed to overcome the geographic and bureaucratic obstacles that perpetuate a debilitating cycle of homelessness experienced by individuals who are undomiciled and suffering from a mental illness, an addiction, and/or a chronic medical condition.

Network Structure

Project WIN functions through partnership agreements approved by HUD; all participating organizations are freestanding, nonprofit, community-based organizations. Although there is no official "board" of the network, there is a formalized structure to monitor and assure that the work of the network continues according to the approved statement of work. Each participating organization contracts to provide a certain array of services as specified in their agreement.

Three standing committees have been established to assist the network in its operations:

- *Executive Committee / Quality Assurance.* This committee meets quarterly and interprets grant deliverables, provides oversight for progress on the grant goals and objectives that are reported to HUD, and oversees operations and fiscal requirements.
- *Supervisor's Operations Committee.* This committee meets monthly to plan and execute the implementation and coordination of services.
- *Shelter Interdisciplinary Team.* This group consists primarily of staff from the four homeless shelters who meet to discuss case-specific issues of the shelters' programs.

These active working committees are essential to ongoing success in the network. They involve key personnel from the various agencies and foster a sense of ownership of the process for all the partners.

All network partners participate in active data collection to track outcomes. Data collection is completed through a Homeless Management Information System supported by HUD. Each of the partners has identified measurable goals to meet within the agreement and data to collect. Beyond the requirements of the grant, these data provide valuable information on the clients, including

- an accurate, unduplicated count of homeless persons who seek services in the region;

- accurate demographic information of the region's homeless population;
- the frequency with which the services are requested;
- the services an individual is currently, or has previously, obtained;
- longitudinal tracking of services provided to an individual; and
- the service and housing patterns of clients within the continuum of care.

The following are core deliverables of the project:

- Seventy-five (75) percent of homeless persons who become engaged in behavioral health services (mental health and/or substance use) will be able to maintain their eligibility for emergency shelter.
- Twenty-five (25) percent of homeless persons enrolled in Project WIN will be linked to housing by the end of the grant period.
- Twenty-five (25) percent of homeless persons identified in the shelter as being eligible for Project WIN (persons with a medical condition, mental health issue, substance use disorder, and/or developmental disability) will engage in case management services.
- Fifty (50) percent of homeless persons enrolled in Project WIN will secure and/or increase their income through either employment or entitlement benefits.
- Forty-five (45) percent of homeless persons completing the Project WIN health assessment with an identified health concern will follow up with a referral to a primary care setting.

The four participating homeless shelters are the focal points for service delivery. Rather than having clients travel to clinics for services, service personnel travel to the shelters.

Eighty (80) percent of the funding for this partnership agreement is provided by the HUD agreement. This totals $1.1 million per year for each year of the agreement and covers the services listed in the project agreement. This is a service agreement; no capital expenditures are allowed. Specific dollar allocations are outlined in the individual partnership agreement. A 20 percent cash match is also required, so other funding streams must be secured and the cooperating agencies must put in funds of their own to meet the Federal requirement.

Membership

Seven nonprofit organizations and CCDPH constitute the network. In the past there were other members, but they no longer participate.

Geographic Area

The service region for this network includes southern and western neighborhoods of Chicago.

Staffing

Administrative staff for Project WIN are provided by CCDPH. Direct service staffs work for their employing agency and are assigned to provide particular services at the homeless shelters as part of their work duties. For example, South Suburban Council on Alcoholism and Substance Abuse provides one full-time addiction counselor to work onsite at the various homeless centers, providing addiction counseling and other services for those clients with an addictive disorder. That employee travels to the various locations.

Range of Services

Through Project WIN, a focused array of services addressing the needs of mentally ill, substance-abusing homeless adult, including persons with developmental disabilities, is made available.

- Shelter
- Care coordination
- Comprehensive assessment
- Mental health services, including onsite assessments, counseling services, psychiatric referrals, medication management, respite care, and crisis intervention services
- Addictions treatment and recovery services, including detoxification, inpatient treatment, halfway houses, and community-based outpatient services
- Primary health care services, including medical prescriptions, and coordinated health prevention services (e.g., flu shots, vaccinations), disease detection (e.g., HIV/AIDS testing, tuberculosis screenings), sexually transmitted disease (STD) testing, and prenatal services
- Entitlement and disability benefits assistance
- Emergency dental/oral services
- Eye exam and eyeglass referrals

Collaborative Efforts

Project WIN is a highly collaborative effort to bring together a more comprehensive service array to a targeted population. Collaboration helps to improve access and engagement in services, and as a result of collaboration economies of scale have been created. Collaborations for specific projects such as this are an economical way to fulfill the intent of these projects. Through collaboration, there is access to a wider array of services. This is beneficial not just to clients but to staff who come in contact with an interdisciplinary cadre of primary and behavioral health care professionals.

Workforce Development

Workforce development efforts do not play a major role in this program other than the network serving as a convener of a broader team to serve a population of adults with multiple problems.

Strengths of the Network

- Project WIN is an engineered network where specific community agencies are brought together to provide an expanded service array for a targeted population and to reduce access barriers to these services.
- Roles of network members are clearly defined through written partnership agreements.
- Standing committees guide the operations of the network.
- Direct service staff go to the client and provide site-based services.
- Difficult-to-treat clients are better served; services are higher quality and are provided in a more coordinated fashion.

Challenges of the Network

- Establishing this network required matching funds by participants.
- Staff turnover at operational levels of providing services challenged service continuity.
- There were challenges setting measurable goals.
- The fiscal agent became the default leader.

Considerations in Forming a Network

The leadership of Project WIN was asked to describe what they viewed as important considerations in forming a network. They identified the following considerations:

- Know your partners.
- Build on collaboration and minimize competitiveness in membership.
- For this type of network, complementary members work best. Complementary members are defined as programs that offer a range of noncompeting and necessary services and supports that help to expand the array of supports to the person served.
- Access nontraditional sources of funding. For example, the Substance Abuse Prevention and Treatment (SAPT) Block Grant and Medicaid are more traditional payers of services. HUD is but one example of a source of funding that would not be seen as a traditional source of funding for substance use disorders.

Looking to the Future

Commitments, formal obligations, and partnership agreements between agencies led to successes and positive outcomes that should continue into the future.

Case Study 4: Maine—Maine Juvenile Treatment Network

Data Sources

- *Interview:* David Faulkner, Executive Director, Day One, Inc.
- *Interview*: Pam Marshall, Director of Prevention and Intervention, Day One, Inc., and Program Manager for the Maine Juvenile Treatment Network

Organizational History

The Maine Juvenile Treatment Network (MJTN), initiated in 1996, is a funded program that coordinates a statewide system to identify, screen, and refer adolescents with substance use issues to participating substance use treatment providers. MJTN is a supported and coordinated effort of the Maine Office of Substance Abuse, Single State Authority (SSA), the Maine Department of Corrections, the Maine Juvenile Drug Treatment Courts, local law enforcement, substance use and mental health treatment providers across the State, other community agencies, and the public schools. The network is operated and supported through a contract from the Maine Office of Substance Abuse to Day One, Inc., for approximately $350,000. Day One is a 501(c)(3) nonprofit, community-based prevention and treatment agency in Portland.

MJTN is not incorporated as a 501(c)(3) entity. The network is a contract of Day One, which serves as the fiscal and managing agency. Day One strives to operate this program with neutrality, maintaining a focus on the overarching goals of improving access and coordinating assessment and referral for adolescents with substance use disorders.

As MJTN has grown and changed over the 12 years, it has increased in both number of providers and number of referral sources. From its beginning with relatively few providers, MJTN now has 54 member providers with multiple members in all regions of the State. In the early years, nearly 100 percent of the referrals were from the juvenile justice system. More recently, the number of referrals from schools across the State, parents, and other sources has increased. The network screens and refers approximately 1,000 youth annually.

The network is viewed as a highly valuable resource in the State because it provides a central place for screening and referral; proactively works to reduce barriers to service; assures that the providers possess the programmatic competencies that are needed to effectively serve an adolescent population; and participates in activities to build the capacities of the adolescent treatment system.

Mission, Values, and Vision

The network's goal is to expand the capacity of the State to effectively treat adolescents with substance use disorders and enhance this continuum of care for juveniles. In addition, MJTN offers support and facilitates collaboration statewide among the Department of Corrections, the Maine Office of Substance Abuse, community-based organizations, school personnel, and treatment providers.

MJTN facilitates regular communication, meetings, and training addressing a variety of issues, including case-specific problems/issues, best-practice approaches to treatment, communication and information sharing, identification of gaps in and barriers to treatment services, and other community issues.

MJTN uses the following global strategies to ensure success of this program:

- Identify youth who have a problem via network partners, including juvenile corrections officers; teachers, guidance counselors, or principals at local middle schools or high schools; local law enforcement; and parents.

- Provide a standardized screening/assessment tool (Juvenile Automated Substance Abuse Evaluation [JASAE]) to identify whether or not further service is needed.
- Maintain an extensive database of qualitative and quantitative data based on JASAE to inform decision making for service delivery and fund distribution.
- Refer youth to a local network substance use provider member.
- Ensure that providers maintain professional integrity of licensing and certification standards.
- Ensure that the provider offers a sliding fee scale for clients.
- Ensure that potential barriers for treatment are eliminated to the extent possible.
- Provide funds for treatment when a child does not have private insurance and does not qualify for Medicaid (i.e., be the "payer of last resort").
- Provide funds for transportation if needed.
- Provide incentives and benefits to become a member and part of the MJTN team.
- Provide opportunity for provider networking.
- Provide continuing education opportunities for members via conferences and workshops.
- Provide opportunities to give feedback on MJTN policies and procedures via an advisory group.
- Disseminate information to the community.

Network Structure

MJTN is a collaborative effort of member organizations and other interested agencies that provide screening, treatment, referral, and other services for substance-affected juveniles (under the age of 18) throughout the State of Maine. When the network was first implemented, very few agencies in Maine were providing services for adolescents. This funding to support network and capacity building was seen by the State agencies as a method to engage more agencies to provide treatment for substance-affected youth. Member agencies were encouraged and supported to participate in the network through positioning MJTN as the "payer of last resort" for adolescents and as a payer for services that would not customarily be paid for by traditional funding sources, including transportation and childcare. Currently 54 agencies are involved. Additionally, 50 high schools are engaged, along with juvenile corrections officers and other community service organizations.

Funding for Network

MJTN is primarily funded through a sustaining contract for $337,396 for services covering the entire State of Maine. Approximately 25 percent of the funds are allocated for treatment and complementary services. The bulk of funding is allocated to operating the statewide program. Additionally, the network has pursued other competitive funds to support its activities.

Network Governance

It is recognized that MJTN is a contract of Day One and operates within this organization's system and structures. As such the network does not have a formal and truly independent governing board. There is an Advisory Council to provide direction and guidance to the network and its staff. The Advisory Council is composed of representatives from the participating agencies. The direction and input of the council informs and shapes the actions of MJTN.

Membership

To become a participating member in MJTN, agencies complete an application. There is no fee to become a member. Agencies that join MJTN agree to adhere to and maintain certain requirements and certifications required under their membership agreement and contract with the SSA for alcohol and drugs. Agencies must

- be licensed by the SSA,
- be Medicaid eligible,
- provide outpatient and/or intensive outpatient substance use disorders services in one or more service locations, and
- adhere to network policies.

Further, direct service providers commit to the following activities and goals:

- participate in network-sponsored training events;
- attend a minimum of three network meetings in a year;
- incorporate into adolescent treatment programs use of evidence-based or best practices as defined by the network in collaboration with the SSA and supported by research;
- use network-developed protocols and forms for communication between MJTN, network member treatment providers, Department of Corrections, and community organizations;

- collaborate with other network members and participants to identify gaps in services and work cooperatively to fill those gaps;
- participate in a network screening and referral system designed to match client needs with provider strengths and capacity;
- participate in network development of policy, procedures, and training designed to implement network goals and support provider conformance with these goals; and
- complete in a timely manner required SSA admission and discharge forms with the appropriate network coding.

Geographic Area

This program offers services statewide.

Staffing

MJTN currently has one full-time and four part-time staff positions. Staff are primarily involved with screening and referral activities, providing network member services, and supporting network capacity building.

Range of Services

With membership and participation in the network, agencies receive the following benefits:

- *Funding.* MJTN is a payer of last resort for outpatient treatment services available for qualifying youth served by network providers.
- *Training and workforce development.* MJTN provides a range of ongoing training and technical assistance for the purpose of building the overall competence and effectiveness of the adolescent treatment workforce in Maine. Participation in training is free for network-sponsored events
- *Initial telephone screening.* MJTN provides initial telephone screening for youth in need of services.
- *Client screening.* The JASAE is administered on a face-to-face basis.
- *Client referrals.* As a participant in the network, members make and receive referrals of adolescents in need of assessment and treatment services.
- *Client support.* MJTN assists clients in reducing access barriers to services.

- *Needs assessment and systems capacity building.* There is input into the development of network policy and a system of comprehensive care for adolescents.
- *Data collection and analysis.* A comprehensive database has been created for data extracted from the common assessment form completed by all clients. Providers contribute to data collection and data analysis. These data are used for systems improvement through identifying gaps in and barriers to treatment services throughout the State.
- *Networking and communication.* MJTN hosts regular meetings to facilitate communication between referral sources and treatment providers.

Collaborative Efforts

Through the collaborative efforts of MJTN, a network of treatment providers with special expertise in working with adolescents has become operational. Through this network, cross-systems collaboration with education, juvenile justice, and other youth-serving organizations is improved. Collaborative efforts also support regional and statewide data collection, analysis, gaps identification, adoption of evidence-based practices, and ongoing efforts for systems improvement.

Workforce Development

The development of a trained and competent adolescent treatment workforce is a high priority for MJTN and has been since its inception. A number of workforce development initiatives have been supported by this program.

- *Assessing workforce training needs.* Through its Advisory Committee, network provider meetings, and other sources, MJTN gathers information identifying current and emerging training needs.
- *Providing training.* Training is supported through MJTN resources.
- *Implementing and adopting evidence-based practices.* The MJTN has supported providers to build capacity for implementing youth specific evidence-based practices.
- *Requiring best practices.* All agencies participating in the network agree to evidence-based and/or best practices as part of the contractual arrangement the network has with the State Office of Substance Abuse.

- *Facilitating communication and network among providers.* Many providers in this State exist at a distance from other providers. The network provides a platform for providers to come together in a collegial environment to interact and exchange ideas. This peer-to-peer collegial support has been a valued by-product of this collaboration.

Strengths of the Network

- The treatment provider system is highly invested in the network because the network addresses multiple needs by being a payer of last resort, a payer of services not usually funded by insurance, a source of training that is reflective of the providers' identified needs, and a source of networking among colleagues.
- The network has been a successful vehicle to build statewide capacity for adolescent services.
- The network provides an identified statewide resource to assist referral sources in placing adolescents.
- The network sets standards of care for their treatment provider membership.
- The network supports the adoption of best practices and evidence-based practices for serving adolescents.
- The network uses a common screening tool across the system.
- The network has developed IT capacity to collect data about youth and families served and to use this information in planning and improving service delivery.
- The network is viewed as a real and successful model of collaboration and partnership among community agencies and State youth-serving agencies.
- The network is viewed as a highly affordable model that could be replicated and could have similar benefits of building systems capacity to serve youth or even other populations.
- The network provides collective advocacy for addictions treatment issues.

Challenges of the Network

- Recently, there have been growing concerns in the network that school systems are moving away from "social and restorative models" and moving toward a more punitive interpretation of the "zero tolerance" substance use policy; with the latter policy, adolescents found using substances are expelled from school rather than being referred for evaluation and services. Concurrent with this trend has been a reduction in federal funding for Safe and Drug Free Schools school-based programs.

Considerations in Forming a Network

The leadership of Day One and MJTN were asked to describe what they viewed as important considerations in forming a network. They identified the following considerations:

- Have the State agency be a partner and funder of the network.
- Create an environment where providers can build collaborative (not competitive) relationships; building collaborative partnerships among members is viewed as "key."
- Develop infrastructure that is responsive to the needs of the population served and the network membership.
- Develop database capacity for client services, management, and long-term planning.
- Have a reliable common screening tool that can be used for screening and referral, provider communication, client services, data collection, analysis, and planning.

Looking to the Future

Areas of future growth for the network include

- better engaging community referral sources that have historically underutilized the network, with a goal for these referral sources to more consistently use the network;
- seeking out additional resources that would allow the network to expand its capacity to deliver expanded "wraparound" types of services for youth;
- exploring the expansion of this type of collaboration, which is currently unique for adolescent services, to the adult population; and
- diversifying the base of network funding. Currently, the network is dependent on State grant funds for its operations. Diversification would not only allow for expansion but also build a stronger financial base (sustainability) in case of State funding reductions.

Case Study 5: Massachussetts—Behavioral Health Services Network

Data Sources

- *Interview:* Peter Lenrow, Executive Director, Somerville Mental Health Association
- *Other sources*: documents and the Web based materials

Organizational History

Somerville Mental Health Association (SMHA), the lead agency in the Behavioral Health Services Network (BHSN) in Somerville, was founded in 1964 by a coalition of parents, school administrators, and the Massachusetts State Department of Mental Health. SMHA was established in response to Federal legislation that funded community mental health centers across the country and was part of a decentralized behavioral health system being established to serve Somerville and Cambridge. This decentralized system includes private, not-for-profit agencies in the area providing supportive housing, substance use disorders treatment, and a range of community mental health services. SMHA has always operated as part of a system of collaborating providers.

The agency is a functioning community mental health center. Its largest population consists of adults with severe and persistent mental illness, and over 60 percent of agency clients experience co-occurring substance use disorders.

BHSN was also founded in the mid-1960s, through the efforts of SMHA. This network was born out of a commitment to quality care through collaboration among diverse agencies. BHSN has made it possible to provide more comprehensive services to people with a range of mental illness, substance use disorders, and co-occurring disorders.

Mission, Values, and Vision

The primary mission of SMHA has been to meet the behavioral health needs of people who live or work in Somerville, giving priority to those with low incomes and other underserved, socially marginalized persons. To address these needs, SMHA provides both preventive and clinical services designed to "enable individuals to experience greater competence and social support in the least restrictive environments and to promote respectful and supportive qualities in community life that can nourish such healthy changes." SMHA serves children, families, and individual adults.

The philosophy underpinning the network is very consistent with systems of care principles and values (Child Welfare Information Gateway, 2008). Within this framework, local agencies partner with families and communities to address the multiple needs of persons and families involved in the systems. At the heart of the effort is a shared set of guiding principles that include interagency collaboration, individualized strengths-based care, consumer involvement, community-based services, and accountability. The interagency collaboration created through the network reduces barriers, improves access to services, and aids in coordination of efforts.

Network Structure

This network is an informally organized coalition of more than 24 nonprofit community-based programs who provide an array of services in mental health, substance use disorders, homelessness, primary health, early childhood education, suicide prevention, and youth crisis. BHSN has developed over the years as a resource and referral network through which clients have access to a wide range of services. It is the intent of the network to be somewhat invisible or seamless in appearance to the clients. With a coalition structured in this manner, many of the elements of a formal network are not present. Each agency maintains its own board, budget, policies, and procedures. A memorandum of understanding exists only with the four public or quasi-public agencies participating in the network:

- Massachusetts Department of Public Health, Bureau of Substance Abuse Services
- Massachusetts Department of Mental Health, Metro-Boston Area
- Cambridge Health Alliance (psychiatric emergency services for Somerville)
- Somerville Court Department of Probation

The network agencies have a wide range of relationships with each other, ranging from a “handshake agreement” to formal contracts for services.

The network has launched a Web site, www.somervillementalhealth.org, to serve as a resource guide to assist potential clients, providers, and the public in finding services in the area. The site describes all mental health, substance use disorder, and co-occurring disorder services available in the community (within the network) and provides the information needed to refer a client to any agency within the network. The network of providers itself is largely invisible to the client. Service providers within the network primarily use other network members when there is a need for other levels of care or other collateral services. To facilitate this process, SMHA is adopting a standardized comprehensive assessment tool that eventually will be used with all clients, both at intake and then approximately 6 months later to gauge the effectiveness of treatment. For clients in need, SMHA has the capacity to provide case management services to aid the client in navigating the network and accessing services. Additionally, SMHA holds several State contracts that allow the purchase of targeted client services from providers within the network.

Legal Structure

The network is not a formal legal entity such as a 501(c)(3) nonprofit or an incorporated membership association. There are no elected officers and no designated staff for the network. Communication activities and network support are primarily provided by SMHA staff. The executive director of SMHA functions as a spokesperson for BHSN.

Membership

Network members include a wide range of community nonprofit service providers who serve clients in the Cambridge/Somerville area.

Geographic Area

BHSN serves the Cambridge/Somerville area.

Staffing

Designated staff positions are not dedicated to BHSN activities. The SMHA executive director is the identified spokesperson for the network and takes the role of convener of BHSN meetings and facilitator of communications among members.

Range of Services

The services provided by BHSN can be described within two frameworks: (1) services that support providers in the network and (2) services available to consumers within the community. A common Web site is used to inform and guide potential service recipients and provides a place to exchange information, share resources, and collaborate. Further, shared resources are available for training. The network participates in the ongoing assessment of service needs for the community. In the absence of a common data system within the network, this needs assessment process is mostly anecdotal and qualitative. For consumers of services, the network offers a broad array of clinical treatment, primary health care, and other complementary services that are often needed by a behavioral health treatment population. The network helps to reduce access barriers and improve coordination for consumers.

The following services are provided by the network:

- *Community mental health services:* outpatient assessment, psychotherapy, psychopharmacology, community rehabilitative support, case management, day treatment, assertive community treatment, substance use and dual diagnosis treatment, family crisis intervention, hospital-based and mobile psychiatric emergency services, and inpatient assessment and treatment
- *Health promotion:* Early Head Start and Mental Health Consultation, Head Start, early intervention, pediatric care, and oral health services
- *Family recovery services:* services for substance-abusing parents and/or adolescents requiring treatment and documented abstinence in order to be reunited as a family
- *Homelessness prevention:* community outreach, case management, and housing assistance
- *Suicide prevention:* support groups for parents, siblings, and close friends of youth who have died by suicide or overdose
- *Somerville youth crisis response network:* a collaboration among the Somerville Health Department and trained crisis workers from multiple agencies and community volunteers

Collaborative Efforts

There are noteworthy collaborative efforts of the network. First is the previously described Web site, where services and access to service are described in a manner that is client driven. Second, services are delivered by multiple entities in an informal manner. The third effort, which is under way, is the development of a common assessment tool to be used across providers.

Workforce Development

- A principal workforce development activity of this network is shared in-service education opportunities.
- Enhanced communication and collegial contact among providers have developed.
- Training is available using shared resources

Strengths of the Network

- This network is truly a grassroots community effort to build and support a network of service providers. It exists largely through the in-kind contribution of staff time and other resources, without formal structure and with little funds from outside sources.
- The network brings together behavioral health, primary health, housing, education, child care, and other social service organizations.
- The network includes providers of services, payers, and State licensing/ regulators.
- Through collaboration, innovative and expanded services are available to the community.

Challenges of the Network

- The absence of formal structures for the network, including an identifiable business entity, staffing, data systems, and strategic planning processes, limit the scope of activity that can be accomplished.
- The absence of resources to support the network infrastructure limits membership services, including enhanced workforce development activities.
- The scarcity of overall resources hinders network development.

Considerations in Forming a Network

The Executive Director of SMHA was asked to describe what he viewed as important considerations in forming a network. He identified the following considerations:

- Assess the needs within the community.
- Identify how your organization and others can respond to those needs.
- Assess the readiness and willingness of providers to collaborate in forming a network.
- Involve clients in identifying how the network should benefit the clients.
- Identify how the network would benefit the participating organizations.

Looking to the Future

Future goals for the network include plans to initiate a common psychosocial assessment among participating agencies.

Case Study 6: Nebraska—Touchstone

Data Sources

- *Interview*: Jason Conrad, Executive Director, Houses of Hope, Lincoln
- *Other sources*: organizational documents and Web-based materials

Organizational History

This collaborative program began in 1997 between two nonprofit agencies in Lincoln: the Houses of Hope and CenterPointe. Both are well-established residential programs for adults ages 19 and older. One agency, Centerpointe, primarily serves a mental health population and the other agency, Houses of Hope, serves an addictions population. In the late 1990s, the State regional center providing substance use residential services was closing, and the State decided to redistribute these beds according to their historical allocation formula across the six mental health regions of the State. A Request for Proposals (RFP) was posted by the State, and Houses of Hope decided to bid on the RFP.

In responding to the RFP, Houses of Hope proposed to implement a program with integrated co-occurring disorders capacity. To this end, they approached CenterPointe about a partnership in this proposal and the resulting program. The two agencies had a history of cooperation and were located within a few miles of each other. CenterPointe had complementary service capacities that Houses of Hope did not have at that time, namely nursing, psychiatry, and medication management. CenterPointe readily agreed to be part of the RFP, and the Touchstone program was born. The State funded the proposal for Touchstone, and services began shortly after that.

Today Touchstone is a highly structured short-term residential substance use and co-occurring disorders treatment facility for adults, offering individual and group counseling, psychotherapy, psychiatric consultation, medication management, nursing, and case management. Touchstone treats patients with chemical dependency and co-occurring disorders through a 12-step facilitation and cognitive/behavioral therapy orientation to treatment. Beyond the acute treatment phase, Houses of Hope provides a range of community-based treatment options plus intensive care management and supportive housing. The program and this collaboration are now in its 11th year providing services in the Lincoln urban area.

Mission, Values, and Vision

The Houses of Hope programs provide quality affordable residential treatment services to individuals in recovery from substance dependence.

Network Structure

Touchstone remains under the corporate umbrella of Houses of Hope and has not separately incorporated as a nonprofit agency, though the two founding partners are both 501(c)(3) nonprofit agencies.

Since Touchstone began in 1997, the two agencies have operated under the terms of a written contract with the State of Nebraska Department of Health and Human Services. This contract is renewed annually. The two agencies have developed a joint Memorandum of Understanding (MOU) that has been in effect from early 1999 and has 2-year renewal cycles. This MOU defines duties, tasks, and responsibilities of each partner, which are described below.

While both Houses of Hope and CenterPointe maintain their separate boards of directors, Touchstone has a Project Management Committee comprised of staff members from each agency to provide day-to-day oversight for the collaboration. Overall program administration and oversight is provided by the Touchstone Advisory Committee, comprised of two board members from each organization, as well as the executive directors of both agencies and the clinical director from CenterPointe. The Project Management Committee recruits, selects, and supervises the director of the Touchstone program, who, in turn, supervises the staff dedicated to running this 24-hour-a-day service. Though the Project Management Committee does not have public members or consumers on the committee, feedback is obtained through voluntary satisfaction surveys completed by residents and family members of the residents.

Part of the unique nature of this collaboration has been the ability of both agencies to assess and capitalize on their strengths and provide services accordingly. To that end, the two agencies have assigned responsibilities for the administrative functions of Touchstone according to their respective capacities. Houses of Hope serves as the fiscal agent and provides office staff support. CenterPointe coordinates data collection for quality improvement and program evaluation. The agencies share in the provision of clinical services, with Houses of Hope providing counselors, technicians, and an office assistant and CenterPointe providing the program director, a case manager, a recreational therapy assistant, medical staff, and a cook. Funding through House of Hope is allocated so as to support this shared staffing model.

Membership

The Touchstone collaboration is between two organizations; Houses of Hope and CenterPointe. Both agencies are 501(c)(3) nonprofits with facilities in Lincoln.

Geographic Area

This program primarily serves a defined service region in Nebraska, but it has the capacity to serve clients statewide.

Staffing

This program uses a highly creative co-located staffing model, but staffing challenges have occurred. To address these issues, a joint management infrastructure was developed.

As issues of administrative/organizational structure between the two agencies emerged, the Touchstone Advisory Committee studied the issues and made recommendations to the boards of the agencies so that the issues could be resolved jointly. Staffing for the program was accomplished through a joint agency hiring process, regardless of which agency ultimately employed the staff member. The overall management infrastructure was built around collaboration and shared decisionmaking.

Range of Services

Touchstone provides a 22-bed (9 females and 13 males) short-term residential program (average lengths of stay 30-45 days); one of the beds is dedicated to referrals from the Indian Health Center. On average during a year, the program treats approximately 175 clients. Of the 22 beds, the State contract funds 18. The remaining beds are contracted to other purchasers, including Medicaid and vouchers from State Probation and Parole Office.

Program components include

- intake assessments and diagnostic services;
- individual services planning, reassessment, and discharge planning;
- individual, group, and family counseling;
- nursing and medical services, including psychiatric consultation and pharmacological services as needed;
- case management services;
- community / daily living skills training;
- recreational therapy services;
- crisis response services;

- an introduction to self-help programs; and
- followup postdischarge.

The primary source of funding for this network is the State contract. Additional funding streams have been added over the years. Medicaid now covers a small portion of clients, and the State Probation and Parole Office provides vouchers for services. The program is at maximum capacity for clients at most times, with waiting lists of up to 6 months.

Collaborative Efforts

This program showcases the benefits and some of the challenges of collaboration. Through the collaboration of two organizations, a new program has been created that would have been beyond the individual capacities of either individual partner. Collaboration is demonstrated throughout the program model, program staffing, management, and administration. The creation of the joint management structures is identified as core to the infrastructure making this program successful.

The work atmosphere created at Touchstone has been described as very positive, and the program has enjoyed almost no turnover in staff; many clinical staff have been employed for a number of years. It is thought that this stability is partly due to these structures that support planning, problem solving, and staff development.

Workforce Development

A number of innovative workforce development initiatives are identifiable in Touchstone:

- Shared staffing is a cornerstone of innovation in this program.
- Developing a successful joint management infrastructure has enabled this program to problem solve issues as they occur and has built cohesion within this program.
- Staff professional development is a value within the organization. Staff for Touchstone provides support so that staff can become dually credentialed as both mental health providers and licensed alcohol and drug counselors. All credentialing and re-credentialing fees are paid by the network.
- All training events that staff attend for both initial credentialing and renewal of credentials are paid for by the network. The program contributes to college education costs.

- A common understanding of the program and its components has been created by a common language among staff.

Strengths of the Network

- Through collaboration at all levels of the program, these two agencies have demonstrated true synergy: the two coming together have been able to create something that neither individual party could have created alone.
- The creation of a shared management structure is viewed as central to the strength and success of the program.
- An integrated model for the treatment of co-occurring disorders is provided through collaboration.

Challenges of the Network

- Developing a common language and common vision for the program is an investment of time and resources.
- Collaborative decisionmaking can be time-consuming and at times cumbersome. No unilateral decisions are made. All decisions go through a process that might involve both parent agencies and both boards.
- Adequate funding is always a challenge in public programs.
- In the past, staffing challenges included
    - program staff coming to Touchstone from differing philosophical and clinical approaches,
    - developing a unified approach to treatment,
    - developing protocols for new staff hires,
    - developing program policies and procedures across two agencies, and
    - a number of human resource issues based in different agency practices.

Considerations in Forming a Network

The leadership of Touchstone was asked to describe what they viewed as important considerations in forming a network. They identified the following considerations:

- Work out as many of the management details in advance as possible.
- Create forums for discussion and problem solving.

- Look carefully at the mission and culture of your partners to see if they are complementary.
- Seek to create equality between partners in decisionmaking, program development, operations, successes, profits, and losses. The convergence of interests and commitment will be crafted through heated dialog, but this dialog ultimately brings out the best of each agency to create a positive and real commitment to the mission and goals of the venture.
- Collaborations can occur with many agencies or between just two.

Looking to the Future

Staff of Touchstone report that sometimes success breeds its own challenges. The program is heavily utilized and nearly always has a waiting list for services. They have begun the exploration for larger quarters.

There have been discussions of a merger from time to time between Houses of Hope and CenterPointe. To date the two agencies have not determined that merger is the best avenue for them, although each entity brings particular strengths to the table, which makes a merger seem more desirable. The agencies are committed to their programs and value the unique cultures of their organizations. They do not see the need or value for the creation of a "mega-agency" in their region.

Case Study 7: New York—North Country Behavioral Healthcare Network

Data Sources

- *Interview*: Barry Brogan, (founding) Executive Director and CEO, North Country Behavioral Healthcare Network
- *Interview*: Lowell Warner, Director of Membership Services, North Country Behavioral Healthcare Network
- *Other sources*: organizational documents and Web-based materials

Organizational History

North Country Behavioral Healthcare Network (NCBHN) was incorporated in December 1997 as a 501(c)(3) nonprofit, tax-exempt organization, following several years of cross-agency collaboration in a rural region of northeastern New York State. NCBHN covers the six upstate New York counties of Clinton, Essex, Franklin, Jefferson, Lewis, and St. Lawrence.

A rural area, these six counties on or near the Canadian border have a combined total population of just 450,000 (in a State of over 19 million) and span more than 200 square miles of territory. The initial motivation that brought this group together was the perceived challenges of a managed Medicaid system being implemented in the area. It was the belief of participating organizations that collaborative efforts would provide support in infrastructure development, assist with potential economies of scale, and overall provide a competitive advantage within a managed care payer environment. The participating agencies that formed NCBHN collaborated to investigate various network models they might adopt as a region, thus giving them more negotiating power with potential managed care companies.

At about the same time, the New York State Department of Health launched the Rural Health Network (RHN) Development Program. The purpose of the RHNs was (and is) to help rural communities strengthen their health care systems through networks or partnerships by the integration of administrative, clinical, financial, and technological functions across their organizations. These RHN programs were supported by the State to help reduce fragmentation of health care services in rural areas, improve coordination of services, and achieve economies of scale. The State provided up to $150,000 per network to support startup and establishment as an RHN. A successful application was filed for one of these grants by the newly formed NCBHN; the application emphasized a unique strength of linkage between behavioral health care and primary health care. The initial grant monies from the State commenced in early 1998, and NCBHN became staffed and operational at that time. Managed Medicaid services were never implemented in this region because it was determined that the small population and rural nature of the area did not lend itself to a successful implementation of managed Medicaid products. Despite this change, the participating network members viewed the network as valuable and have continued to do so to this day.

With the initial incorporation of the network and the establishment of a modest dues structure, concerns emerged among the public sector (State and county) agencies that had been part of these initial operations. Anecdotally, it was reported that the public agencies withdrew from the network citing concerns for potential conflict of interest. These public agencies, in addition to providing some direct services, saw themselves as charged with certain regulatory, enforcement, and program funding obligations. Additionally, several nonprofit organizations decided not to join because of the fees associated with membership.

Today, the network members provide an array of services for adults, adolescents, children, elderly people, and Native Americans. Services are provided in the following areas: primary health, mental health, developmental disabilities, substance use disorders, temporary housing, prevention, education, and advocacy. Behavioral health care services span the continuum from acute inpatient services to community-based outpatient and recovery supports.

In 2001, the North Country Management Services (NCMS) LLC was formed as an outgrowth of NCBHN to provide an array of business products and services, including: management consulting, IT services, accounting services, administrative support, training, event management, project management, grants development and administration, employee benefits, and group purchasing. NCMS is co-located at NCBHN headquarters and is staffed by network employees. NCMS is owned and managed by network members and serves the dual purposes of providing a range of business services to network members (and others) for a fee and generating income for the network.

The network is supported through a variety of sources including a variety of grants, membership dues, income generated by NCMS, and fees.

NCBHN remains an open system and accepts new organizations as members. The network provides its members with a level of communication, collaboration, and regional advocacy that has positioned network providers to shape and influence emerging behavioral health care policies and practices, particularly those that impact service quality and access. In addition to the shared voice the network brings its members, it also offers its members many tangible services that will be described later in this case study.

Mission, Values, and Vision

The network has clearly articulated statements of mission, values, and vision:

- *Mission:* NCBHN connects and supports behavioral health providers to strengthen the service delivery system in northern New York.
- *Values:* NCBHN is committed to and accountable for achieving excellence through collaboration and builds on the mutual trust, respect, and values of its partner organizations.
- *Vision:* NCBHN will be widely recognized as a leading voice for northern New York's behavioral health care continuum, bringing the necessary resources for the connection of advocacy efforts, technology development, and best practices among partners.

Network Structure

Legal Structure

NCBHN is an incorporated 501(c)(3) nonprofit membership organization; it currently has 20 active members. As framed in the organizational bylaws, there are nine board members who can be elected from the executive directors / CEOs of the member organizations. All board members and board officers have term limits so that over time all member organizations will serve as board members for the network. Officers of the board are elected by board members. The board maintains a highly active and influential system of committees in which all NCBHN members participate. Committees are actively engaged in assessing community need, planning, implementation of specific projects, and evaluation. Quarterly, there are full meetings of all NCBHN members where plans and performance of the network are reviewed and discussed and where current or emerging needs in the community are identified. There are currently six positions in the network, including the CEO.

The board and the staff rely on the strategic plan, now in its fourth iteration since the beginning of the network to determine the direction of the network. To make sure the strategic plan is followed, the board president and the executive director hold a conference call regularly that is dedicated to evaluating adherence to the strategic plan. In addition, elements of the strategic plan are now included with the annual contract with the State.

Committee Structure

NCBHN has an active and involved committee structure, including an executive committee and committees on membership services, strategic planning, assessing community need and strategic planning, special project management, and quality improvement.

Membership

There are currently 20 organizational members in the network. Eleven members provide a range of addictions treatment and recovery services and mental health / psychiatric services. Four organizations are youth-and family-serving organizations. There are three prevention programs, two health centers, and one advocacy organization for persons with serious and persisting mental illness. Membership in the network is highly stable.

Members enter into a contractual agreement when joining the network and agree to pay annual dues ranging from $250 to $1,000. Each member has one vote, regardless of organizational size. A high level of commitment is expected from the member organizations. The CEO or executive director must be the board representative, or if the CEO has sent a person in his or her place, that person must be vested with sufficient authority to vote on binding network matters. Other member organization staff can participate on committees as might fit with their expertise and interest.

Geographic Area

NCBHN covers the six upstate New York counties of Clinton, Essex, Franklin, Jefferson, Lewis, and St. Lawrence. Some limited services have been provided outside of these counties, but no member organizations have sites outside this geographic area.

Staffing

Currently there are four full-time and two part-time employees, as well as consultants as needed. The CEO/ executive director, director of member services, office manager, and financial manager are full-time positions; the IT specialist and the project specialist / training coordinator are part-time positions.

Range of Services Provided by NCBHN

- Organizational capacity building, particularly in areas related to information technology and electronic records implementation
- Facilitation of collaborative efforts
- Advocacy at the State and Federal levels
- Community needs assessment and planning
- Public education and outreach
- Individual member services
- Training and workforce development

Range of Services Provided by NCMS

NCMS offers business products, business management services, and IT support to members and non-network members. Currently the most actively used services are accounting and IT services, followed by training, benefits services, and group purchasing of materials and supplies. Training is offered through conferences, classroom training, and online/Web-based learning. Grant management services that include prospecting, writing, and managing are also offered. Services are described in more detail below.

Management Consultation

- Executive transition
- Operating policies and procedures manuals
- Cost reduction / profit improvement
- Business and marketing plans
- Operational analysis / process improvement
- Organizational change/restructuring
- Fraud detection and recovery

Accounting Services

- Bookkeeping: Providing computerized bookkeeping services using QuickBooks and Peachtree, for use at the member's office or remotely
- Payroll: Providing payroll services in conjunction with bookkeeping services or separately; includes preparation and filing of all payroll tax reports
- Audit preparation: Preparing annual audit and audit report
- Financial controls: Designing policies and procedure that can help alleviate the possibility of fraud and waste in the organization; additionally, reviewing books and reconciling bank accounts on an ongoing basis as part of a plan of assurance that accounts are being properly maintained
- Accounting software implementation: Installation (by certified QuickBooks Pro Advisors) of QuickBooks or Peachtree software in the organization and providing training and support for staff

Information Technology

- IT support services: Administration, maintenance, and support on a weekly basis to help organizations maintain and support applications, backups, network connectivity, servers, users, security, and workstations
- Strategic and implementation services: Development and enhancement of IT strategy to reach business goals
- Infrastructure and network services: Identification of needs and a project plan that will lead to implementation
- Project management
- Overall grant project management
- Tracking project timelines and milestones
- Meeting management
- Reporting

Transition Management

- Analyzing and documenting the duties of a staff position
- Temporarily performing the tasks related to the position
- Training new hires
- Supplementing staff skills with temporary or ongoing assistance

Employee Group Benefit Plans

- Medical
- Dental
- Life insurance
- Vision
- Statutory disability insurance (under New York State's Disability Benefits Law [DBL])
- Disability
- 401(k) retirement
- Voluntary benefits

Collaborative Efforts

The network currently facilitates a number of collaborative programs and initiatives. The role of the network varies depending on the specific initiative, ranging from facilitating collaboration among network members to developing "cooperative agreement" grants, serving as the lead and fiscal agent for the grants, and grants management.

Children's Mental Health Initiative

The Children's Mental Health Initiative is a collaborative effort by network members in Essex and Franklin Counties to expand access to children's mental health services in the region. The initiative was funded in 2003 though the Federal Health Resources and Services Administration (HRSA) Office of Rural Health Policy. Strategies pursued as part of this initiative have included efforts to recruit a board-certified child and adolescent psychiatrist to provide services in the counties, placement of a school-based mental health worker in the school district serving St. Regis Mohawk Reservation students, and development of a telepsychiatry program in Franklin County schools and the clinics serving the two counties.

Fort Drum Regional Health Planning Organization Behavioral Health Committee

The Behavioral Health Committee is one of four committees formed by the Fort Drum Regional Health Planning Organization (FDRHPO), a not-for-profit corporation recently formed in Jefferson County, New York. This committee is part of a U.S. Department of Defense pilot program that is exploring the feasibility of building cooperative health care arrangements between military installations and local nonmilitary health care systems. Staffed by NCBHN, the FDRHPO Behavioral Health Committee focuses on planning and evaluating the provision of behavioral health care service to Fort Drum military personnel, their families, and residents of the communities surrounding Fort Drum.

North Country Network of Care for Behavioral Health

The North Country Network of Care for Behavioral Health is an initiative that created a Web-based "Network of Care" for Essex, Franklin, Jefferson, and St. Lawrence Counties in northern New York. Each county Network of Care Web site provides individuals, families, and care providers easy online access to information about mental health, substance use, and developmental disability services in the region. NCBHN is providing data collection and verification services and technical assistance to the community services directors at the four county sites since 2007.

Northern New York Technology Alliance

The Technology Alliance is a group of 13 NCBHN members working to develop a HIPAA (Health Insurance Portability and Accountability Act of 1996)–compliant Integrated Advanced Information Management System (IAIMS). Also known as a Health Information Technology System (HITS), the system will improve quality and increase access to care by sharing critical clinical data between behavioral health providers (including mental health and substance use services) and primary care physicians, clinics, and hospitals. HRSA's Office of Rural Policy recently awarded the Technology Alliance (through NCBHN) grant funding to move forward with development of this initiative.

Points North Housing Continuum of Care

The Points North Housing Continuum of Care is comprised of representatives of more than 50 agencies and faith-based groups as well as individuals concerned with meeting the needs of the homeless and those at risk of homelessness in Jefferson, Lewis, and St. Lawrence Counties. The group recently received funding for two initiatives: the Shelter Plus Care program and the Homeless Management Information System (HMIS). The Shelter Plus Care program offers qualified Jefferson County residents (disabled persons, including those with mental health and/or substance use problems) a rental voucher for up to fair market value if the client agrees to accept other in-kind support services available to them, including health care, child care, education support, and case management. HMIS is a Web-based database that will allow participating providers to collect data on the homeless and access information about resources available throughout the region. Ultimately, HMIS will help the Points North Housing Continuum of Care to develop a more accurate view of the severity of the homeless problem in northern New York, and to maximize resources available.

Tri-County Pathways to Balanced Nutrition

A volunteer coalition of school and community health professionals joined together in 2004 to address the need for early assessment and treatment of eating disorders among students in Jefferson, Lewis, and St. Lawrence Counties. To date, the coalition has engaged in community outreach and education, developed clinical expertise, and established a case management program to help families navigate the system. They have also developed a partnership with Strong Memorial Hospital in Rochester for expert case consultation, including telemedicine and clinical supervision, for NCBHN mental health and primary care providers. The network has provided financial, staff, and logistical support since the project's inception.

Workforce Development

NCBHN has been credentialed by the State of New York as a substance use training provider. They have crafted core curricula to train clinicians preparing to become certified substance use counselors, and they provide continuing education for credentialed providers. They also have a cooperative agreement with an organization that provides online courses. The training capacity of the network has helped to develop a more skilled and credentialed workforce in the region and has aided in workforce recruitment in a geographic area that has workforce shortages. Training through the network also provides opportunities for formal and informal networking among clinicians, which it is hoped will aid in workforce retention. The network also assists with recruitment of workers through advertising (primarily); for some positions the network staff will prescreen candidates. The network is just beginning to explore a possible role in facilitating job sharing, particularly for positions such as psychiatrists that are very hard to recruit.

Strengths of the Network

- The network has maintained a high-quality professional staff with significant nonprofit business management expertise.
- Network staff demonstrate a high level of membership service (customer service).
- The network has developed an organizational culture where organizations can come together in a noncompetitive and collegial environment benefiting from peer-to-peer interactions.
- The network has the capacity to facilitate collaborative ventures among members.
- The network provides multiple venues for members to provide formal and informal input into needs assessment and planning processes.
- The network has a governance structure that is highly responsive to member needs.
- The network has a high level of commitment and involvement among member organization senior leadership.
- The network has a proven track record and consistent support from the State.
- The network offers an array of services that support the business infrastructure as well as professional development for the direct service workforce.
- NCMS not only provides useful and important business services to members, but it also generates revenue for the organization.

Challenges of the Network

- The biggest challenge identified by the organization is its overreliance on grant dollars to support the infrastructure and operations of the organization. They are hopeful that NCMS will continue to grow and provide increasing revenue to the organization.
- Although the membership has been stable for a period of time, increasing membership in the network would enhance its collective influence and provide further opportunities for service and collaboration.

Considerations in Forming a Network

The leadership of NCBHN was asked to describe what they viewed as the most important consideration in forming a network. They identified the following considerations:

- Incorporate democracy into the operations of the organization.
- As quickly as possible, incorporate and establish a recognizable identity.
- Charge dues to build a sense of ownership.
- Senior leadership of member organizations must be involved.
- Move away from having a fiduciary agent as soon as you are able.
- Regularly assess needs of your members and of the community you serve.
- Provide the best membership services you are can.
- Allow the members to set the agenda.
- The organization must be responsive to the needs of the members.
- In the governance policies have "one member one vote," term limits on board officers, and multiple ways for members to provide input.

Looking to the Future

Staff of the network is extremely optimistic about the future of the organization. It has a solid foundation of service to its members and continually assesses the needs of members and the community through its members. They are engaged in what they believe are a number of highly important initiatives that are of value to the members and to the network. Most notably, they are working with providers to develop and successfully implement electronic patient records and build stronger linkages between behavioral health care and primary care.

Case Study 8: North Carolina—Guilford County Substance Abuse Coalition

Data Sources

- *Interview*: George Coates, Executive Director, Guilford County Substance Abuse Coalition
- *Other sources*: organizational documents, Web-based materials, and IRS Form 990 for 2006 and 2007

Organizational History

The Guilford County Substance Abuse Coalition (GCSAC) is an incorporated 501(c)(3) nonprofit founded in 2002. GCSAC is a coalition of organizations providing prevention and treatment services for substance use and mental health disorders, including local government, hospitals, physicians, social service providers, public schools, colleges and universities, libraries, law enforcement, community organizations, and faith-based organizations.

GCSAC was formed following a health conference held in May 2002 at Guilford Technical Community College near Greensboro. This event mobilized community leaders to recognize that substance use disorders are matters of serious public health concern in Guilford County. Recommendations growing out of the event called for

- a community coalition to be formed to study the issue,
- assessment of available resources and gaps in services, and
- establishment of a system for ongoing planning of services and monitoring of services and community needs.

GCSAC emerged at a time when the State of North Carolina was undergoing a radical transformation of its mental health and substance use disorders service delivery system. Previously most services had been provided by public State and county agencies. Sweeping mental health reform was under way in the State, and most services were being privatized. This change provided both impetus and opportunity not just in Guilford County but also across the State to begin new programs, because many clients would be transitioning from public programs to private sector programs financed by Medicaid and the SAPT Block Grant funds. To build a responsive community-based system of care, it was essential to assess service delivery capacity and gaps, and GCSAC became the agent for that assessment in the community.

Early in its formation GCSAC was a recipient of a SAMHSA Drug Free Communities Grant to support its development. Subsequently GCSAC membership became actively involved in Community Anti-Drug Coalitions of America (CADCA), a 501(c)(3) nonprofit organization that works to strengthen the capacity of community coalitions in their effort to create and maintain safe, healthy, and drug-free communities. CADCA supports its members with training and technical assistance, public policy advocacy, media strategies, marketing programs, conferences, and special events.

GCSAC was formed by representative stakeholders and individual citizens of Guilford County, an urban county in north central North Carolina. GCSAC established five standing committees to begin the work of the coalition: steering, needs assessment, best practices, monitoring and planning, and community awareness. Members were drawn from local service providers and community residents. The Moses Cone–Wesley Long Community Health Foundation and the Community Foundation of Greater Greensboro provided funding to GCSAC, and the coalition hired an executive director.

From that initial group of 40 agencies and individuals in 2002, GCSAC has nearly doubled its membership. Today there are 72 members, including organizations and community members. Given the size of the membership and its policy and commitment to inclusion, GCSAC decided to establish a 15-member board of directors to help with the workflow.

The founders of GCSAC believed a network should be diverse and inclusive and should support comprehensive approaches to treatment and prevention services, using evidence-based practice to integrate substance use and mental health disorders treatment with primary care. This comprehensive approach and improved integration could be supported by increasing the coordination and effective utilization of community assets and by addressing the gaps between treatment programming based on traditional unit-based State and Medicaid funding categories and the needs of persons affected by substance use disorders. GCSAC recognized the limitations of traditional treatment systems and sought to increase the array of longer term recovery support services, including housing and supportive programming options.

Mission, Values, and Vision

Mission Statement

The coalition brings together the provider community and Guilford County residents to develop a partnership through advocacy, education, collaboration, and support of best-practice principles to effectively address substance use.

Civic and community leaders and GCSAC members felt that GCSAC should be a long-term alliance between providers, schools, social services agencies, public services agencies, and the community as a whole. GCSAC goals would be to

- establish and maintain a stable and functioning coalition;
- conduct a comprehensive community substance use needs assessment that includes an inventory of community resources and identification of gaps;

- encourage and support the implementation of best-practice principles for substance abuse prevention, treatment, and aftercare programs;
- establish and maintain an ongoing monitoring and planning of service system; and
- build community awareness of substance use disorders through social marketing, education, and advocacy.

Network Structure

GCSAC is an incorporated 501(c)(3) nonprofit organization with 72 active organizational and community members. An elected board of directors is nominated from GCSAC's membership. Membership to GCSAC is an open-enrollment process; the only requirement is either being a resident of Guilford County or doing business in the county. The organization receives funding through several grants and has an annual budget of approximately $175,000.

The original board was formed from the Steering Committee, but now the board is elected through a process by which a Nominating Committee, composed of the committee chairs, brings forward names to the board on an annual basis. The Nominating Committee seeks a cross-representation of the community. Terms for board membership are for 3 years, with one-third of the board rotating off annually.

In addition to the Nominating Committee, GCSAC currently has committees on needs assessment and monitoring, education and training, community awareness and advocacy, finance, and steering.

As with most new organizations, establishing an organizational structure and increasing membership were important early goals. To guide their efforts, GCSAC developed a strategic plan. Within the current strategic plan, the following four objectives are the areas of focus:

- Develop an organizational structure.
- Establish and maintain a planning and monitoring system.
- Raise awareness about GCSAC.
- Promote best practices.

Membership

GCSAC currently has 45 organizational members and 27 community members. Organizational members include representatives from local government, social service providers, substance use service providers, mental health service providers, hospitals, libraries, and community organizations, schools, law enforcement, and faith-based organizations. The community members include individuals and business representatives.

Geographic Area

GCSAC primarily services Guilford County but also participates in some statewide planning efforts.

Staffing

GCSAC has two paid staff positions: an executive director and a support staff position. Committees and other activities rely heavily on volunteering coalition members.

Range of Services

- *Maintaining an active and engaged coalition of community stakeholders.* To support this effort GCSAC holds regular coalition meetings, prepares and distributes a quarterly newsletter, conducts community forums, and participates in a broader coalition of nonprofit service providers.
- *Facilitating.* The primary role of GCSAC is *not* one of direct services; rather, it facilitates community mobilization, planning, and implementation of services for the county.
- *Assessing substance use service needs for Guilford County.* GCSAC contracted with a consulting company to complete a community assessment and draft a written report for distribution. A survey was developed and completed by more than 500 persons representing a broad base of input. Aggregate data were studied, and a published report assessing community substance abuse needs with accompanying recommendations was completed in 2005. This document has been widely distributed and has been used by county planners and service providers to assist with planning activities. To sustain the ongoing efforts of community needs assessment, GCSAC has a standing Needs Assessment and Monitoring Committee.
- *Supporting the adoption of evidence-based practices.* GCSAC has funded and hosted a number of training events for the adoption of specific evidence-based practices for providers, including Solution Focused Therapy (SFT); Life Skills Training (LST); Screening, Brief Intervention and Treatment (SBIRT); and Motivational Interviewing (MI). These training events have been offered at no charge to local

providers. Further, GCSAC financially supported the delivery of LST to sixth graders in county schools.

- *Building community awareness.* GCSAC has conducted multiple activities to build community awareness regarding substance use, prevention, treatment, and recovery.
- *Supporting targeted efforts for prevention of substance use among youth.* GCSAC has conducted a number of youth-specific activities, including funding LST, hosting a youth substance abuse summit, educational activities at high schools and colleges, and supporting a range of other youth activities.
- *Disseminating information.* The coalition serves as a clearinghouse of substance use information in the county. GCSAC publishes a quarterly newsletter and has created a community resource directory for Guilford County. The resource guide includes listing and contact information for all substance use and mental health resources, other social service organizations, 12-step groups, and other self-help and recovery support groups.

Collaborative Efforts

A fundamental principle of GCSAC is to facilitate collaboration within the county for the planning and delivery of quality substance use services that are responsive to the unique needs of this community. Collaboration is evidenced in the organization's makeup, with broad-based stakeholder membership. GCSAC's collaboration with service providers includes supporting their efforts in planning appropriate services and adoption of evidence-based practices. GCSAC membership has been enlisted to provide education and training for the members and the community. In 2006, for example, GCSAC provided SBIRT and MI training. Lastly, GCSAC collaborated with the Guilford County corrections system to create a reentry program for persons leaving the county corrections facility.

Workforce Development

GCSAC was created to give a voice to community stakeholders as co-planners in the development of this new system in North Carolina. Beyond planning and development activities, GCSAC has played a more targeted role in training and the adoption of evidence-based practices. The creating of the community resource directory also was described as an important aid to staffing.

Strengths of the Network

- The network was created with broad-based community representation to support capacity building for substance use services, including prevention, intervention, treatment, and recovery support services.
- The network is inclusive of both organizations and individuals.
- The network plays a key role in the community, assessing needs for services.
- The network provides a neutral forum where diverse interest groups can come together and build consensus on strategies to address community needs.
- The network is a support and advocate to the provider network.

Challenges of the Network

The following challenges have been identified:

- Ensuring the network would not become too provider heavy and lose some of its broad-based stakeholder focus
- Maintaining the commitment and the enthusiasm of members
- Avoiding turf conflicts between providers over limited resources
- Sustaining resources to support operations

Considerations in Forming a Network

The GCSAC leadership was asked to describe what they viewed as important considerations in forming a network. They identified the following considerations:

- The total community should be involved because addiction is a total community issue; no one segment of the community can solve it alone.
- To sustain a coalition such as this, members require continued support and motivation to remain involved, and, ultimately, members must believe that their efforts are making a difference in their communities.

Looking to the Future

The leadership believes that one of the major accomplishments of GCSAC is that the organization helped shape services at the community level during the rapidly changing environment of mental health reform in North Carolina. Three major commitments for the future are efforts to improve access to services for persons in need, providing ongoing support to providers adopting and implementing evidence-based practices, and continuing to assess community needs.

Case Study 9: Oregon—Oregon Treatment Network

Data Sources

- *Interview:* Bruce Piper, Oregon Treatment Network
- *Other sources*: organizational documents, Web-based materials, and IRS Form 990 for 2006 and 2007

Organizational History

In 1995, the State of Oregon announced a plan for a Medicaid redesign. The redesign possibilities included a managed care option, rebidding of Medicaid contracts, and other options that could place smaller providers at a disadvantage. The possibility of these changes brought five substance use service providers together to form a statewide network, the Oregon Treatment Network (OTN). It was their belief that forming a network could give provider members an improved ability to approach any statewide or regional payer from a position of greater strength. Contracting with OTN gave these providers the ability to cover the entire State or any of its regions.

Ultimately, Oregon did not implement a Medicaid managed care option, as was originally discussed. Beyond the original motivation in forming the network, members saw inherent value in continuing its operation and have expanded and redefined its goals and services during the past 12 years. Today OTN is primarily a network of providers for the treatment of substance use and co-occurring disorders serving central Oregon.

OTN became a 501(c)(3) nonprofit organization in 1998. The corporate entity of OTN serves as a fiduciary agent for a series of grants for network members and provides other member services. OTN is a closed member system; unless there is an identified unmet need within their system, OTN does not solicit new members.

A full continuum of substance use treatment services are provided through the network, spanning all levels of care. Additionally, OTN provides a range of specialty services, including integrated co-occurring disorder treatment; intensive adolescent outpatient and residential treatment; specialized women's and children's programs; Latino/Hispanic programs; agonist therapy, including methadone treatment and buprenorphine; DUI programs; smoking cessation;

life skills development; relapse prevention; transitional housing; permanent drug-free housing; childcare; and problem gambling treatment.

The network provides services at all levels of clinical care across most of the State in rural, suburban, and urban communities. It serves all age groups and has specialized programs for youth and women with children. It also has the capacity to serve diverse racial and linguistic groups.

The network has positioned itself uniquely by creating common quality assurance and quality improvement protocols across the system to establish a certain level of uniformity in processes and a capacity to collect and analyze data both within an individual organization and across the system.

Mission, Values, and Vision

OTN brings together and coordinates the efforts of five nonprofit treatment and prevention organizations in central Oregon. With 100 years of collective experience, OTN provides quality substance use prevention, intervention, and treatment services that are more comprehensive and diverse and cover a wider geographic area than any single provider in Oregon. Timely access to services, commitment to quality care, and services offered at a reasonable cost to payers are values of the network.

Network Structure

OTN is a 501(c)(3) nonprofit. To maintain the work of OTN, there is a small governance structure. There has been an ongoing decision by the OTN board to not grow the OTN infrastructure and to pass the resources that would have been used for growth on to the members. The executive directors of the member agencies serve as the board of OTN under its bylaws. Staffing of the network is provided by the member agencies. The network funds two part-time positions: an accountant and a legislative liaison.

The network has an annual budget of $2.4 million, primarily from grants. Annual dues are paid by each member in the amount of $5,000. In addition to the member dues, OTN retains 1 percent of each contract to support administrative costs of the network. Since nearly all of the grant monies are passed through to member agencies, if a particular grant requires a higher level of administrative activity this function is subcontracted to one of the member agencies.

The network has both standing and ad hoc committees, including an executive committee, a legislative committee, quality improvement, and training.

Membership

Membership in the network has been based on a number of considerations, including location, service region, and service array. Five members are in the network.

Geographic Area

OTN provides services statewide.

Staffing

Staffing of the network is largely provided through in-kind services from its members. There was an early decision made in creating the network to not invest significant resources in program infrastructure costs. The two part-time positions are paid by the network, and if grants call for higher levels of administrative support these functions are subcontracted to the members.

Range of Services

Membership Services

OTN provides a number of services, including marketing of membership services, serving as a fiduciary agent on contracts, supporting cross-organization collaboration and cross-systems quality improvement activities, and legislative advocacy. OTN has managed a number of training contracts that have benefited the members and other providers.

Clinical Services

Through the network membership a full array of clinical services for adults and youth with substance use and co-occurring disorders is available, including treatment, intervention, and prevention. Treatment services include detoxification, outpatient, intensive outpatient, methadone maintenance, residential, and intensive residential. The network also provides specialty services, including transitional housing, day care, transportation, specialized outpatient, intensive outpatient, and residential treatment for women, adolescents, adult corrections clients, and dual-diagnosed clients. Though all of these services are not available in every OTN location, they represent a diverse continuum of services available from one source in the State.

Each OTN member follows specific quality assurance procedures, which are standardized across the system. Each OTN member has a long history of excellent clinical performance as measured against the Oregon Administrative Rules (OARs) that are the State standards of care governing the delivery of services. Client Satisfaction Questionnaires (CSQs) indicate that 93 percent of clients felt very positive about their treatment and 90 percent of them would return in the future if necessary; 83 percent were pleased with the timeliness of the services rendered.

Participation in the National Institute on Drug Abuse Clinical Trials Network

A unique capacity of the network is its ability to participate as the community treatment provider system for the National Institute on Drug Abuse (NIDA) Clinical Trials Network (CTN) conducted through the Oregon Health Services University. The mission of CTN is to improve the quality of drug abuse treatment throughout the country using science as the vehicle. CTN provides a platform in which NIDA, treatment researchers, and community-based service providers cooperatively develop, validate, refine, and deliver new treatment options to patients in community-level clinical practice. OTN participates in this endeavor as its members provide treatment sites across the entire State of Oregon. Their participation also helps them increase and improve the quality of their evidence-based practices.

OTN's participation in CTN is based on their capacity to span multiple service-related domains, including diversity of clientele (in age, gender, and racial and linguistic groups) and type of community (rural, suburban, and urban); their capacity for cross-site collaboration; and their capacity to generate a sufficient cohort of clients for the research projects.

Collaborative Efforts

There are a number of noteworthy collaborative efforts within OTN.

- There is a high level of interagency collaboration in the delivery of client services.
- There is collaboration between network members on quality assurance and quality improvement practices.
- There is interagency collaboration on grants.
- There is interagency collaboration on staff training.
- There is collaboration with NIDA CTN. The CTN effort is simplified by working with one entity that spans multiple domains of service, geography, and populations.

Workforce Development

OTN has managed various training contracts over the years to provide training for the staffs of the member agencies. Through their contractual involvement with CTN, clinical and program staff have enjoyed a rich opportunity to be a "greenhouse" for evidence-based clinical practices. Staff enjoy close working relationships with practice developers and researchers, including high-quality implementation training, supervision, and coaching that supports high levels of implementation fidelity. Further, representatives of OTN participate in CTN advisory workgroups helping to facilitate a "science to service" and "service to science" dialog.

Clinical staffing within OTN is described as highly stable. In part, this speaks to the stability of the organizations, but it also speaks to the clinically and intellectually rich environment in which practitioners work.

Strengths of the Network

- The network offers all levels of clinical care.
- The network spans most of the State, serving rural, suburban and urban communities.
- Minimal competition exists within the network because network members have geographic service regions.
- The network spans all age groups and has specialized programs for youth and women with children.
- The network has the capacity to serve diverse racial and linguistic groups.
- The network has created common quality assurance and quality improvement protocols across the system.
- The network has a close working relationship with a major research institution that is a source of revenue and a rich source for staff professional development.
- The network is a conduit of revenue for members.
- The network supports governmental and legislative liaison and support for members.
- Peer-to-peer sharing, support, and problem solving is an extremely valuable aspect of the network.
- The strong "state-of-the-art" clinical programs of OTN provide a competitive advantage to the network with regulators and payers of services.

Challenges of the Network

- OTN does not maintain an open enrollment practice for new members. It is recognized that competitive relationships with other non-network agencies in the State exist.
- Changes in State funding strategies are a continuing concern. Oregon has adopted a system of "Home Rule Charter" for counties where planning and funding for services is increasingly directed by locally elected county planning boards. The county boards are obligated to formulate written plans for substance use services. The counties have the option of contracting out services or delivering those services directly by county employees. There are concerns that Home Rule Charter approaches do not interface as easily with networks. This type of county purchasing system curtails the degree to which the network will grow.
- The large geographic area of the State creates access problems for network members to frequently meet face to face. This has been ameliorated by use of technology.

Considerations in Forming a Network

Network leadership was asked to describe what they viewed as important considerations in forming a network. They identified the following considerations:

- Pick your partners very carefully.
- There must be real value created through the network for it to survive. Too many coalitions are formed where a structure is created that just perpetuates itself and does not really provide any value either to programs or to persons served.
- The relationships among members should be complementary and supportive.

Looking to the Future

OTN leadership advocates for the State to have a role in helping alleviate perceived issues and limitations created through county-based purchasing. They support the creation of incentives for communities or regions developing local networks for substance use disorders services. They believe that private providers are more agile and more able to effect program changes and implementation in a timely manner.

Another concern looking to the future for the network centers on the aging of its senior leaders. There are concerns that the next generation of leaders may not share the same vision of the power and benefit of networks.

SUMMARY OF CASE STUDY FINDINGS

Networks have existed in health care for decades and have been a growing presence in behavioral health since the 1960s. The importance of networks and collaborative relationships became part of public behavioral health policy dialog with the introduction of "systems of care" in mental health services (http://www.systemsofcare.samhsa.gov/). Interest and at times urgency toward forming networks has been driven by State- and national-level changes in the payer system, increased reporting demands, and rates of reimbursement that have not kept pace with costs of doing business. Many States have moved away from historic grant and aid contracts to fee-for-service models that require further changes in the infrastructure of organizations, including changes in staff roles and organizational structures and the need for more sophisticated information systems. Networks were viewed as strategies to remain competitive in the marketplace, create economies of scale, share resources, and create a stronger voice in State agency and legislative processes.

Another and equally important driving force in network formation is the actual patients served in a program. Clients entering the publicly funded treatment system have multiple problems (CSAT, 2007). In fact, most patients experience problem-saturated lives. The formation of networks enables providers to better create a continuum of care and within that continuum a richer array of services at all levels of care. These networks can improve access and retention, improve coordination of care, improve team approaches to service, enhance collegial input, and create rich opportunities to train and develop the workforce.

Types of Networks

In this study, five of the nine networks have become freestanding 501(c)(3) nonprofit corporations. Boards of directors are drawn from network membership in CAARR, CFBHN, NCBHN, GCSAC, and OTN. Three networks have an agency serving in a role as the lead and fiduciary agent

(Project WIN, MJTN, and Touchstone). BHSN is a coalition of providers that have come together in a loosely formed coalition to cooperate as they serve patients.

Network Services

Network services to membership span a full range of options and appear to be largely determined by the needs and the interests of the participants.

- *Provider network management:* defining continuum of care and the service array; determining the types, number, and qualifications of providers based on community needs; selecting providers; credentialing; ongoing communication with providers; and training and technical assistance to providers
- *Strategic planning for network:* needs assessment, gap analysis, setting measurable goals and objectives, developing action plans and plans to monitor and evaluate, and community and regional planning
- *Shared quality improvement / quality management:* focus on enhancing access to care, coordination of care, quality of care, efficient use of resources, risk management, and monitoring of State-mandated outcomes. Quality improvement includes ongoing performance improvement initiatives that are based on data.
- *Financial management:* regulatory compliance, grant coordination, proper accounting safeguards, analysis of utilization and cost data, rate setting, claims processing, member services, quality improvement activities, and reporting.
- *Information management:* client tracking, including admissions, authorization, and continued stay; integration of assessment and service-planning data; supporting "seamless" transitions across levels of care; claims management; aggregate reporting; outcomes and utilization analysis
- *Workforce development:* technical assistance, clinical practice development (adoption of evidence-based practices), training, education, and staff sharing
- *Organizational capacity building:* particularly in areas related to information technology, electronic records implementation, improved business practices, and developing new program models
- *Facilitation of collaborative efforts between and among providers*

- *Advocacy at the State and Federal level*
- *Public education and outreach*
- *Accounting services:* bookkeeping, payroll, audit preparation, financial controls
- *Group purchasing:* group benefits plans, program insurance, goods and services
- *Program design*
- *Acting as a fiduciary agent*

Several network practices are innovative and effective. For example, CFBHN has become a provider-governed ASO for the SAPT Block Grant, Medicaid, and other public dollars coming into their region. The network's performance over the years has gained significant attention and admiration because they have consistently demonstrated better-than-average utilization, retention, and outcomes, plus a capacity to creatively configure services to meet patient needs. Their success as a quasi–selfgoverning entity represents a radical alternative to traditional or managed payer systems and at a cost dramatically lower than the administrative fees of most managed care companies. The State of Florida is planning to replicate this model statewide.

CAARR has become the management entity for other small programs. Through this process of shared administrative, fiscal, and supervisory functions, these small programs strengthened and survived, while maintaining their individual program identity.

Touchstone is the smallest network described in this report. Two local agencies came together to form Touchstone, a short-term residential treatment program. These two companies successfully co-located staff from each agency to form this third program. They capitalized on their complementary strengths and were synergistically able to create and successfully operate something that neither could do alone.

These three networks are mentioned as examples of creative and new structures that were successful through networks and collaboration responding to contemporary needs.

Commonalities Among Networks

The networks in this study were chosen to showcase diversity. Regardless of configuration, size, or mission, there are commonalities among the networks:

- Successful networks add value to the membership.
- Competition among providers is viewed as counterproductive to the network.
- Networks are highly participatory.
- Collegiality and peer-to-peer networking is viewed as a highly valuable intangible of the network.
- Formal and informal technical assistance is available through networks.,,
- Advocacy is a function of most networks.
- Networks support and promote collaboration among members.
- Workforce issues are common among networks.

Benefits of Networks to Providers

- Networks can aid the survival and sustainability of an organization.
- Networks can provide shared administrative functions across programs.
- Participation in a network provides access to resources that otherwise may be unavailable (e.g., IT resources and technical assistance).
- Networks can provide competitive advantages pursuing grants and contracts.
- Networks can provide advocacy.
- Networks can provide access to funding, collaboration on grants, advertising and marketing, shared staffing, group purchasing, and other economies of scale.
- Networks can provide peer-to-peer assistance.

Benefits of Networks to Communities

- Networks represent partnerships among providers, allied service organizations, and the community.
- Service networks can improve access and coordination of services to persons in the community.
- Networks bring together a broad array of services to support the person in treatment and recovery.
- Networks can improve communication among patients and those organizations involved in services.
- Patients generally have better responses to treatment when care is coordinated and networks provide enhanced opportunities for integrated responses.

- Networks can play a vital role in community needs assessment, gap analysis, and service planning.

IMPACT OF NETWORKS ON WORKFORCE AND WORKFORCE DEVELOPMENT

For this report, workforce development is described as multiple processes related to the recruitment, training, employment, retention, and professional development of the substance use workforce. At the beginning of nearly all the networks described herein, workforce development was a relatively low priority. Responding to marketplace challenges and community needs were at the forefront of what motivated the creation of networks. Over the past decade workforce issues have risen to become major priorities in most networks, and networks find themselves with unique capacities to respond to workforce issues.

Network Infrastructure

Networks have many of the infrastructure elements to support high-quality workforce development, particularly in areas of recruitment, training, professional development, and credentialing. Networks usually have a physical location with meeting space where training can be conducted. Networks also have fairly direct access to the workforce. The value and impact of a training system is directly related to its responsiveness to the needs of the participants it intends to serve. Networks afford rich opportunities to gather direct input from directors, supervisors, and line staff to more accurately understand the functioning competencies and deficits and reasonable learning objectives. Networks provide rich opportunities for expanded training and professional development opportunities, from traditional workshops to more in-depth skills-focused training, coaching, and mentoring.

Recruitment

Although networks play traditional roles in employee recruitment, they also have the capacity to play innovative and creative roles. Traditional roles include advertising, job posting, job fairs, and outreach to higher education. Innovative roles in recruitment were noted in several case studies. For example, there is job sharing of more expensive professional positions, including physician, executive director, accountant, and clinical consultant, across several organizations. Job sharing is either negotiated through the network or facilitated by the network. Another innovative strategy involves the co-location of staff from two or more agencies to deliver services to a common client population. This strategy has enabled certain programs to operate where they otherwise might not and has improved client access to a richer array of services to meet his or her needs.

Retention

Defined strategies for staff retention were not overtly identified in these case studies, but a number of retention strategies can be inferred. The importance of peer-to-peer support and assistance was consistently identified across the case studies. This support aids in restoring and empowering workers and helps to reduce burnout. Clinical supervision, staff training, and professional development activities (including the subsidization of training and credentialing costs) reinforces staff commitment to the agency.

Professional Development

Rich opportunities for professional development are evident within networks. Several networks have been awarded State contracts for staff training, including both classroom and online courses. These include contracts to prepare workers for certification and licensing. Interestingly, one of the networks also hosts one of the State-authorized counselor certification boards. Many networks provide training and education opportunities, and a number of networks conduct implementation training and other services to support the adoption of evidence-based practices. Lastly, networks provide supervisory training, coaching, and mentoring.

RECOMMENDATIONS AND CONCLUSION

Recommendations

The leadership of the networks was asked to describe what they viewed as important considerations in forming a network. Their recommendations can be summarized as follows:

- Clearly define your vision for the organization based (ultimately) on a commitment of services to the community. Impediments to starting and maintaining an association/network are minimal as long as the organizations involved are committed and solidly behind the mission and the implementation model.
- Regularly assess needs of your members and of the communities you serve.
- Identify how your organization and others can respond to those needs.
- Commit to an ongoing process of quality improvement.
- Having the State agency as a partner and/or funder of the network can be a great benefit.
- Identify how the network will be of benefit to the participating organizations.
- Identify the value created through the network.
- Create an environment where providers can build collaborative (not competitive) relationships. Building collaborative partnerships among members is viewed as key to success. It is important to have a mechanism that supports open and productive communication to resolve any issues and differences among providers.
- Develop infrastructure that is responsive to the needs of the population served and the network membership. Create forums for discussion and problem solving. If a program is going to provide a more complex array of services with potential dual relationships, then these issues must have a forum for discussion and consideration.
- Network partners should be selected based on their ability to be complementary and supportive to others in the network.
- Seek to create equality between partners in decisionmaking, program development, operations, successes, profits, and losses. Partners' interests should converge, and there should be a positive and real commitment to the mission and goals of the venture.

- Incorporate democracy into the operations of the organization. Members should set the agenda. Governance policies should specify one vote per member, term limits for board officers, and multiple ways for members to provide input.
- Incorporate and establish quickly a recognizable identity. Move away from having a fiduciary agent as soon as you are able.
- Ensure that senior leadership of member organizations is involved.
- Networks should have access to an IT infrastructure that includes a database capacity to capture client data and information on funding streams. This will support client services, management, long-term planning, and successful program operations.
- Networks can benefit greatly from using a reliable common tool for screening/ assessment, referral, provider communication, client services, data collection, and analysis.

Conclusion

Richly illustrated in this report are varieties of successful networks. Some networks were driven by the availability of public funding to provide a more comprehensive array of services and to improve access and coordination of care to a targeted population. Other networks grew out of shared provider concerns due to changes and perceived challenges in the communities in which programs had historically conducted business. In a world of increasing patient needs and shrinking dollars, providers considered new and innovative methods of staying in business, so they could continue to serve their communities.

Network models provide structure, resources, and supports to help agencies build more effective business and programmatic capacities. Network programs often have increased access to IT resources, opportunities for funding, technical assistance and resources to build business capacities and a stronger workforce, marketing advantages, and improved governmental and legislative presence, to name a few advantages. Clinically, networks support development of continuums of care, expanded service arrays, improved access and coordination, improved staff skills, and the implementation of evidence-based clinical practices. Successful new configurations of business and clinical practices that are responsive to the needs of the patients and communities served have grown out of these networks. These new structures stand in contrast to business as usual, which in many locations struggles to survive.

These successful systems grew out of the dedication, inspiration, and hard work of individuals working to provide quality services to patients suffering from the disease of addiction. The organizations described in this report shared information about their network generously and freely.

REFERENCES

California Department of Alcohol and Drug Programs. (December 2007). *Fact sheet: Social model recovery.* Retrieved from http://www.adp.cahwnet.gov/FactSheets/ SocialModelRecovery.pdf

Center for Substance Abuse Treatment (CSAT). (2005). *Working definition of recovery [and] definition of recovery-oriented systems of care (ROSCs).* Retrieved from http://partnersforrecovery.samhsa.gov/docs/working definitionofrecoveryand definitionofrecoveryorientedsystemsofcare.pdf

Center for Substance Abuse Treatment (CSAT). (2006). *Addiction counseling competencies: The knowledge, skills, and attitudes of professional practice* (Technical Assistance Publication [TAP] Series 21; DHHS Publication No. [SMA] 08-4171). Rockville, MD: Substance Abuse and Mental Health Services Administration. Retrieved from http://www.kap.samhsa.gov/products/manuals/taps/index.htm

Center for Substance Abuse Treatment (CSAT). (2007). *The epidemiology of co-occurring substance use and mental disorders* (COCE Overview Paper 8; DHHS Publication [SMA] 07-4308). Retrieved from http://coce.samhsa.gov/codresources/PDF/OP8Epidemiology10-03-07.pdf

Child Welfare Information Gateway. *Guiding principles of systems of care.* Retrieved September 29, 2008, from http://www.childwelfare.gov/system wide/service/soc/history/principles.cfm

McLellan, A. T., Carise, D., & Kleber, H. (2003). Can the national addictions treatment infrastructure support the public's demand for quality care? *Journal of Substance Abuse Treatment,* 25(2), 117–121.

National Health Law Program. (2006). *Administrative Services Organizations (ASOs): An alternative to mandatory enrollment of individuals with disabilities into managed care.* Los Angeles, CA.

Whitter, M., Bell, E. L., Gaumond, P., Gwaltney, M., Magana, C. A., & Moreaux M. (2006). *Strengthening professional identity: Challenges of the addictions treatment workforce.* Rockville, MD: Substance Abuse and Mental Health Services Administration.

APPENDIX: LIST OF NETWORKS AND AGENCIES

State: California
Network Name: California Association of Addiction Recovery Resources (CAARR)
Network Description: nonprofit membership association
Type of Services: training, technical assistance, management services, counselor
certification, advocacy
Web site: http://www.caarr.org/
Members: 300

State: Florida
Network Name: Central Florida Behavioral Health Network (CFBHN)
Network Description: provider-operated Administrative Services Organization serving
central Florida
Type of Services: managing Federal block grant, Medicaid, and other public behavioral
health funds; regional planning, training, and technical assistance
Web site: http://www.cfbhn.org/
Members: 19

State: Illinois
Network Name: Project WIN
Network Description: network of providers funded by the Cook County Department of Public Health
Type of Services: substance abuse, mental health, and primary health care services; housing; enrollment in entitlement programs
Web site: none
Members: 8

State: Maine
Network Name: Maine Juvenile Treatment Network (MJTN)
Network Description: network of providers serving adolescents with substance use disorders; managed by Day One, Inc., through a contract from the Maine Office of Substance Abuse

Type of Services: screening, assessment, and treatment services; provider training and technical assistance; data collection and systems improvement
Web site: http://www.juveniletreatmentnetwork.org/
Members: 54, http://www.juveniletreatmentnetwork.org/jtnmap.html

State: Massachusetts
Network Name: Behavioral Health Services Network (BHSN)
Network Description: coalition of behavioral health, primary health, housing, and other service providers serving Cambridge and Somerville
Type of Services: primarily mental health, substance abuse, primary health, and housing services
Web site: http://www.somervillementalhealth.org/
Members: 24 nonprofit community based agencies

State: Nebraska
Network Name: Touchstone
Network Description: residential treatment program for persons with co-occurring disorders
Type of Services: integrated residential treatment
Web site: http://housesofhope.com/ ; http://www.centerpointe.org/
Members: 2

State: New York
Network Name: North Country Behavioral Healthcare Network (NCBHN)
Network Description: rural behavioral health care network and membership association
Type of Services: member services, training, technical assistance, management services, grants development, advocacy
Web site: http://www.behaviorhealthnet.org/home.cfm
Members: 20

State: North Carolina
Network Name: Guilford County Substance Abuse Coalition (GCSAC)
Network Description: incorporated nonprofit coalition of substance use providers and a broad range of community programs and other stakeholders
Type of Services: community needs assessment, service monitoring, planning, training and capacity building, information and referral

Web site: http://www.gcsac.org/about.html
Members: 72

State: Oregon
Network Name: Oregon Treatment Network (OTN)
Network Description: treatment provider membership association and service network Type of Services: prevention, intervention, and treatment services; member of the National Institute on Drug Abuse Clinical Trials Network at the Oregon Health Services University, which provides training to OTN staff
Web site: http://www.adaptoregon.org/Otn.html
Members: 5

INDEX

D

G

H

I

J

K

L

M

N

O

T